# voice

# voice

### disability & ability at LOGAN, 1950-2010

By Gene Stowe

Foreword by Rev. Theodore M. Hesburgh, C.S.C.

Corby Books
Notre Dame, Indiana

# voice

disability & ability at LOGAN, 1950-2010

Copyright © 2010 by Gene Stowe

10 9 8 7 6 5 4 3 2 1

Manufactured in the United States of America

Published by
Corby Books
A Division of Corby Publishing
PO Box 93
Notre Dame, IN  46556
(574) 784-3482
www.corbypublishing.com

ISBN: 978-09827846-4-8

*Featured on the front cover from left to right:  Monty Huddleston, Hayley True, KJ Anderson, and Carol Rita Hamil. On the back cover:  Irving Waxman*

# Contents

This book is dedicated to the individuals who taught us
to look beyond disability.
Their belief in potential opened hearts and minds around them.
And their passion was hard to resist.

Once others were touched by the LOGAN experience, they understood
what the founders knew all along—the power of the human spirit
in overcoming barriers.

This story is for all the people of LOGAN and others near and far
who share the vision to see and the heart to embrace
the ability of every person.

Thank you to all who helped write—and to those
who will continue to write—the LOGAN Story.

# Foreword

The 60th anniversary of LOGAN in South Bend, Indiana, is an opportunity both to celebrate the concrete accomplishments of a local institution and to reflect on a national movement. The same impulse coming out of World War II that accelerated the Civil Rights movement for African-Americans also spawned dozens, maybe hundreds, of organizations like LOGAN. Parents in cities and towns across the country came together to provide a new kind of life for their children who had typically been hidden, or worse, in a society that preferred to deny their existence. Like the Civil Rights movement, this initiative has gained remarkable success—but we still have a long way to go for full inclusion and full recognition of our common humanity.

In South Bend, LOGAN has made a significant difference both for the local community and for the University of Notre Dame. For years, LOGAN's building was right across the street from our campus, and students had an easy walk to an opportunity for service that enriched their lives as much as it did the people they helped. This campus is full of kids who come from stable families, most of them. If you've had all the blessings in life, you share it with people. It was not enough to get a scholarship and come here and get the best Catholic education in the world. We've got to take the Lord's words seriously. The Lord said it all in one sentence: "What you do for one of these my least brethren, you do it for me." The habit of volunteering at LOGAN is a deep root of our service tradition that now involves 80 percent of our students. The work isn't just across the street, but around the world, in places like South Africa where we strive to improve the lives of AIDS orphans.

As this book demonstrates, the movement for equality and inclusion for people with developmental disabilities bears striking historical parallels to the Civil Rights movement. The Civil Rights movement made a difference in America far beyond the gains of African-Americans, including the election of a black president within the lifetime of people who were once blocked from the ballot box. African-Americans became the symbol of all who lack equal opportunity, and the new paradigm of inclusion must be for everyone. For me, the work of LOGAN for people with disabilities, the Civil Rights movement, the service to AIDS orphans, and all such initiatives for equality are all of one piece. They're part of a common mosaic of the least of the brethren. The whole thing hangs together. Like all good works, it's a work of God and a work of grace.

The work of LOGAN and the hundreds of institutions like it across the nation is important not only for the people they serve but also for all of us. As you will see in this book, the presence of someone with a disability in a family is an enriching experience for all the family members. The same is true for the presence of those people in our society. LOGAN has made a difference in countless Notre Dame students' lives, and that's just one instance of how inclusion of such people makes all our lives better. By recognizing their humanity, the humanity we share, we become more humane. They may be the last step on the ladder of equal opportunity for everybody. They're the least brethren today.

*Father Ted Hesburgh*

*Rev. Theodore M. Hesburgh, C.S.C.*
*President Emeritus*
*University of Notre Dame*

# Preface

Eddie was there my whole life, my cousin five years older than I, the second child of my father's elder brother, my favorite Uncle Ed. After a Sunday supper of my Aunt Joyce's homemade hamburgers, Eddie and I would play with Sylvester the cat or explore their walkout basement and laundry chute or watch Walt Disney's "Wonderful World of Color."

At some point, maybe around the time I started school, I noticed that I was still growing up, but Eddie wasn't. I was never sure of the source of his disability. His older sister, Sherry, had none, but their younger brother, D.G., who had such severe disabilities that he was eventually institutionalized.

Eddie, even in a bigger body, would always be the sweet, childlike boy I had known from the beginning, everybody's "pal," "Hey, Cousin" at every meeting, without guile and yet with sharp skills of observation, devotion to his routines, and a knack for noticing the line of least resistance as he navigated 60 years at home. He died in November 2009, not very long after his younger brother.

My hunch is that Eddie and D.G. have as much to do with what we Stowes became as anyone else in my life, and for sure they made a huge difference in the lives of hundreds of people with disabilities in their hometown, Gastonia, and their state, North Carolina.

When Uncle Ed went to enroll Eddie in a private kindergarten, the preacher in charge said, "We don't take his kind here." Ed went straight to the public school officials, who knew change was coming in the mid-1950s, and they set in motion a special classroom each for children with physical and mental disabilities. Aunt Joyce's Junior League paid for the teacher training with proceeds from their charity gala.

Ed championed the cause of disability at home and across the state, lobbying for millions of dollars for the Western Carolina Center where D.G. lived, and where Ed would slip away for hours just to sit with him in a rocking chair. His love for Eddie and D.G. made him the great man he is, and his role as patriarch of our family meant that his rare sense of passion and compassion for the weak reaches into all of us.

My uncle was like the parents in South Bend who started LOGAN a few years before he stood up for Eddie, like thousands of parents across the United States who championed their children's humanity and made us a better society. Telling the LOGAN story, for me, fulfills a family calling.

*Gene Stowe*

Gene Stowe

*"A powerful testimony on the role effective advocacy and community play in the lives of people with disabilities. The people of LOGAN have made a tremendous difference. These stories are told beautifully and show how each person makes a difference over these past 60 years, and for the future."*

John Dickerson
Executive Director
The Arc of Indiana

# Prologue

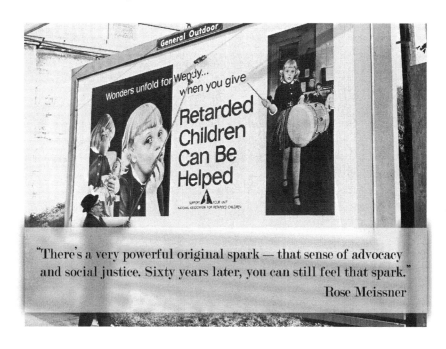

"There's a very powerful original spark — that sense of advocacy and social justice. Sixty years later, you can still feel that spark."

Rose Meissner

# August 1, 2009

From a distance, the celebration at the University of Notre Dame's Stepan Center looks like any of a dozen such summer events in South Bend, Indiana. More than 1,200 people are chatting and hugging and laughing in the sunny field while upbeat music blares from speakers on the makeshift grandstand. Off to one side, huge white tents billow in the gentle breeze, sheltering tables of food and drink that workers set up before dawn. A colorful inflated bounce house and small Ferris wheel stand ready for the Family FunFest at the finish of the sixth annual LOGAN's Run.

Under the balloon-rainbow arching above the start line, Jay Lewis is chatting with Monty while they wait for the starting gun. Jay, a lawyer and LOGAN board member, is running the 10K. Monty Huddleston, a LOGAN client, is aiming for the one-mile walk he's been practicing for weeks with Team LOGAN. Around them, other serious runners go through their stretching routines and don their pedometers amid the happy confusion of participants with cerebral palsy in wheelchairs, entire families with toddlers in tow, children with Down syndrome eager for the fun to begin, casual joggers out for a good cause, teens with autism intent on tracking the course.

At least 50 relatives in the Fonacier family alone shine in bright orange Team Paul t-shirts in support of their son, uncle, brother who brought them to LOGAN. Nearby is a moving sea of blue as members of Team LOGAN—clients, friends, families, and staff—gather in excitement. Team LOGAN, led by the Harris family, carries a sign that reads, "We're Walking the Good Walk Today," a quote from client Terry Harris whose parents, Bonnie and Frank, have long participated in the Adult Day Services parent group.

Race starter Lynn Kachmarik and Jamie McGraw, who has Down syndrome, grow more insistent as the 8:30 AM start time approaches and the racers have to be corralled into position—LOGAN clients leading, friends at their back, a five-minute pause between the Fun Walk that takes its own path and the longer runs around the Notre Dame campus, all rejoining under the rainbow where the start line becomes the finish line.

They're off! The front line clambers forward amid shouted cheers and clapping. Volunteers line the route with printed arrows to guide the runners and cheer them on. Other volunteers staff water stations along the way.

Almost to the finish line, Jay comes upon Monty, who has taken his own leisurely route among the university lawns, and they share a laugh about starting and finishing the race together. The after-run celebration, noisy and colorful, draws curious passers-by onto the campus who discover, on approaching, the uncommon community that has gathered—and the families are welcome to join the fun.

## Sixty years earlier

Maybe Martha McMillian's aunt didn't know the baby, orphaned at only two months old, had disabilities when she took Martha into her home. As she grew, the child earned her keep by cleaning the house, scrubbing toilets, washing dishes, sweeping floors, clearing the table, working in the garden. Maybe Aunt Mary was frustrated by the child's slow responses, so exasperated that she came across mean and harsh, sending Martha to her room. By the time Martha was 8, Mary gave up and sent her to the Fort Wayne State Hospital.

Life for her was no better in the institution. The "slop" offered for food tasted like wallpaper paste or dirt, and, with people crowding the table, she had to use both hands to fend them off and fill her cheeks before the little nourishment would be snatched away. There was an upstairs dormitory for sleeping, a bare-walled first-floor room for sitting, with no organized activity for Martha and the other residents day by day by day. Sometimes they gave her a piece of paper and a pencil and told her to write down her numbers. She took to slipping extra scraps of paper out of the trash cans to sketch the scenes she carried in her mind—churches, homes, trees—a reprieve from the drab environment.

Side by side, these two scenes some 60 years apart suggest a revolution in the relationship between people with developmental disabilities and the larger society. But in South Bend and across the United States, the experience has more resembled an evolution—in its small beginnings, in its incremental stages, in its adaptation to vast changes social and political, educational and economic, medical and technological across six decades, and, perhaps most critically, in its unfinished, ongoing, open-ended development.

That movement began, like so many movements, in the aftermath of World War II, when Americans turned from defeating the horrors of Hitler and saw the reflection of those horrors in their own homeland—assertions of racial superiority, eugenics, depersonalization of those who are different, denial of fundamental human equality and dignity. The same revulsion to such injustice that helped ignite the African-American Civil Rights movement also animated those who championed a new approach to people with developmental disabilities.

The movement challenged a culture that had always hidden people with disabilities in institutions or upstairs rooms—out of sight, out of mind, and out of hope. The movement challenged communities to bring them in, to develop their abilities as well as diagnose their disabilities, to become a society that embraced rather than excluded those with differences in mind or body or both. The movement advanced in parallel with the Civil Rights movement, with individual acts of courage, conviction in the face of community resistance, assists from courts and Congress and presidents. As with the Civil Rights movement, these remarkable gains pose new challenges going forward within a society where it must continue to evolve across generations.

This is a story about that movement—not as an abstract force, but as its flesh-and-blood, bricks-and-mortar incarnation in South Bend known as LOGAN. The movement arose in untold cities and small towns across the United States in the 1950s, largely decentralized even after state and national associations formed a few years after fed-up parents and friends first found each other. Each local expression developed its own character, found its own focus, responded to the specific needs and opportunities in its own place and time. Some, like LOGAN, are celebrating their 60th anniversaries.

Some faded, some flourished, some evolved in different ways. To suggest a "typical" experience, much less a "model," would be misleading. LOGAN's story is not replicated—no one's is—but it will resonate with many of the movement's other incarnations who know the story of their own origins, and with all who share LOGAN's vision for a more fully just society in the future.

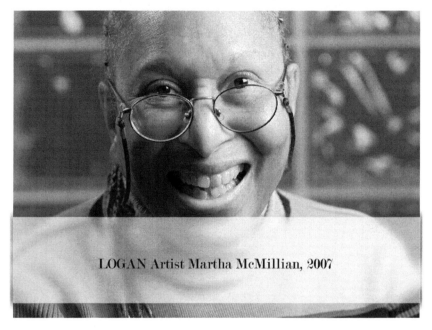

LOGAN Artist Martha McMillian, 2007

LOGAN even wrote a happy ending to Martha McMillian's story. After eight years in the state hospital, when she was 16 years old, Martha returned to her aunt's home in South Bend. When Aunt Mary's health suddenly prevented her from caring for the teenager, she was sent to Plymouth, Indiana, to live and had to do hard sanding in a workshop there.

"LOGAN brought me back to South Bend," Martha said. She lived in two LOGAN group homes and worked at LOGAN Industries, always tidying up her workspace at the end of the day before she retired in 2000. By 2008, she was living in an apartment with a roommate, finally accepting that the staff would do the vacuuming and now, in her 70s, she no longer has to earn her keep.

"I love my apartment," she said. "You can have a whole room of your own. We get to have a bathroom of our own. I like my own bathroom."

Martha has also learned to eat more slowly and confidently, and she still fills journals with penciled multiplication tables. She goes on trips to Chicago with her advocate and friend Sue Correa, shopping at Navy Pier and taking in the play *Mary Poppins*. She'd like to take the train to California some day, and maybe even to visit Washington to meet President Barack Obama, whose achievements make her proud of her African-American heritage.

She takes art, nutrition, exercise, and music classes and watches movies in LOGAN's program for folks her age. Her own art—sometimes drawn on the inside of discarded cereal boxes and slipped under Sue's office door—has won wide acclaim, commissioned among other things for greeting cards from Notre Dame's Athletic Department and Mendoza College of Business.

# chapter 1

# Beginnings

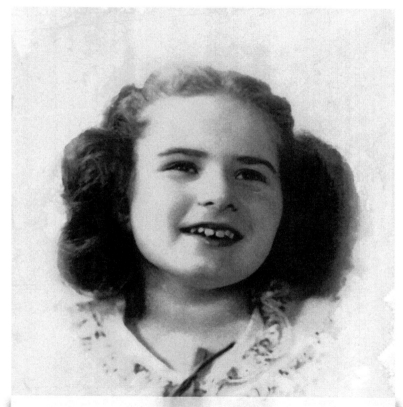

"...you were our motivation, our spirit. Whatever we are today, we are better because you lived, and oh, so thankful that you were ours."

Joseph J. Newman

The doctor told Joe and Sophie Newman to institutionalize their newborn daughter Rita Jo as soon as possible, to avoid the trauma of a later move. An accident with forceps during her birth had left her brain bleeding, and she would be severely disabled for the rest of her life. The Newmans should move on.

Joe knew something about putting people away. His parents were exiled to Siberia by the Czar before the Russian Revolution. Nothing like that was going to happen to Rita Jo. She was still their daughter. They would take care of her.

Joe, a Jewish grocer in largely Catholic South Bend, soon saw the gift that Rita Jo was to his family. He also saw the gift that the rest of society was missing by excluding such people. So he set out to make life better both for those with disabilities and for the community that needed them.

"People were saying, 'Put this child away and have another child,'" he said. "If something was going to be done, I had to do it. I had to sit down and see what I could learn. Then I just went out and started talking."

What he found was a world that looked on people with disabilities as inferior, unworthy, and a potential threat to the vitality of the gene pool—much as many of them thought of African-Americans in an age of anti-miscegenation laws.

"That's the concept that people had," Joe said. "That's what people were taught. The doctors were saying, 'Put your children in an institution.'"

At one point, the Newmans succumbed to the experts' pressure and took Rita Jo to a carefully-selected institution in Montgomery, Alabama, where they would go to see her once a quarter. She stayed for 18 months.

"Every three months we went down, she was weaker," Joe recalled, and the couple decided to bring her home. "With every mile we got closer to South Bend, she got stronger," and she broke into a smile when the family reached the front door. "Don't discount what these kids know. A child can die of a broken heart."

Joe joined the American Association of Mental Deficiency—he was the second member from Indiana—and soon saw that the experts would not lead change. It was up to parents.

"There weren't too many of us," he said. "The public thought they were doing the right thing. They believed it was going to destroy the gene pool."

In newspaper articles printed by a sympathetic editor who had an institutionalized sister and in talks to the Rotary Club and other civic groups, Joe challenged the narrow, Stepford-like notion of "normal" that justified the exclusion of the disabled—and many others—from full participation.

"Any normal society contains abnormal people," he said. "Otherwise, it's not a normal society. You mark the maturing or the growth of a society by how it recognizes the fact that everybody in the community is not the same. If a society is going to mature, it has to have room for these people."

Joe also insisted that parents show the pictures they carried of their children—all their children, even the one with a disability whose picture usually stayed in the back of the wallet. No more out of sight, out of mind, as such children had been for generations. A county school superintendent in Indiana once told Newman that he knew of no such children in his county.

Meanwhile, day in and day out, Joe and Sophie were working to make a life for Rita Jo and living with the nagging question: "If something happens to us, who will take care of her?" Sophie, who had found another family with a disabled child to play with Rita Jo, decided they had to do more.

"One day, Sophie said, 'We can't be the only ones with this problem,' and she went out and found three other women," Joe recalled. "They met. She came home another day and said, 'We started an organization, and you're president.'"

The Council for the Retarded of St. Joseph County incorporated and acquired a dilapidated school building, long used for storage, on the

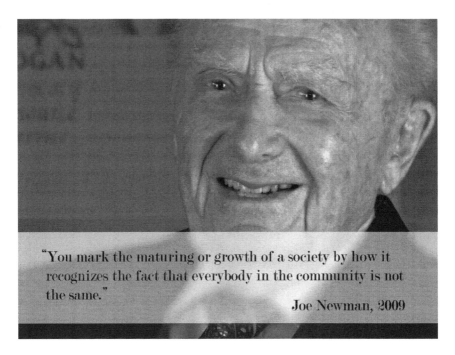

"You mark the maturing or growth of a society by how it recognizes the fact that everybody in the community is not the same."

Joe Newman, 2009

grounds of Family and Children's Center in Mishawaka. Lent to LOGAN by that agency, the building was filthy, bleak, and bare of anything useful for operating a school. Parents pitched in to clean and paint it, bonding in their shared work for their shared concern for their children and their society. Joe heard of a demolition company owner who was tearing down a school in Michigan City and storing the salvage in Cassopolis, Michigan. Despite her reputation as a brusque businesswoman, the owner told him to take whatever he needed for the project. She understood because she had a grandchild with disabilities.

When an inspection by the fire department revealed that the building needed a new boiler, a local plumbing manufacturer donated the equipment and the plumbers' union installed it. The painters' union helped with the painting, and an outdoor sign company installed a large sign next to the bright-white building: "LOGAN School for Retarded Children." No more out of sight, out of mind. LOGAN School opened in 1950 with 22 students, two teachers, and $24 cash.

From that beginning, LOGAN has grown into one of the country's leading centers of services and advocacy for people with disabilities. It has reached into the fields of employment, housing, education, recreation, rehabilitation, guardianship, and protective services. It has lobbied and filed lawsuits on behalf of people with disabilities. It has recruited thousands of college students and community volunteers. It helped host the International Summer Special Olympics Games and launched its own foundation from the profits. It has won the admiration and support of the top civic and governmental leaders in its community, honored, among other things, with the first Leighton Award for Non-Profit Excellence by the Community Foundation of St. Joseph County in 2000.

"LOGAN makes us more enlightened," said Community Foundation Director Rose Meissner. "There's a very powerful original spark—that sense of advocacy and social justice. Sixty years later, you can still feel that spark. LOGAN is operating with the interest of its clients and families first and foremost. I respect and admire how LOGAN has not been eroded or diminished. I think LOGAN makes us better. It's not just what it's doing for its clients and families. It makes the rest of us more decent, more civilized."

From its beginning, LOGAN cut across ordinary dividing lines of race, religion, socioeconomic status, and ethnicity. African-Americans were attending LOGAN School long before the public schools were integrated. Some of the first Asian families in the city found themselves and their children welcomed by the Council for the Retarded. Well-meaning Catholics marveled that Joe, a Jew, was sharing in the good work of Fr. James Smythe, a priest who held parent meanings and seminars promoting education for children with disabilities.

Today, LOGAN serves more than 1,000 families a year, employs more than 350 workers, operates eight group homes, and provides jobs for 160 people in a 90,000-square-foot manufacturing center in an industrial park. Its 40,000 square-foot headquarters on a major South Bend street houses multiple programs and a center for autism, responding to the fastest-growing disability in the nation. Families have moved to South

Bend and business executives have turned down out-of-town promotions so their children can enjoy the life that LOGAN supports.

Although the inspiration for the effort, Rita Jo Newman, who died at home with her parents at her side at age 28 in 1966, never received any services or benefits from LOGAN. Yet her parents, the Council for the Retarded, her northern Indiana community, and all those touched or moved by the ministry for 60 years have benefited from her life.

---

A Father's Thoughts
by Joseph J. Newman
1966

Our daughter Rita Jo died yesterday and to us, just a simple obituary will not do justice. Rita Jo was injured at birth and was a severely retarded, cerebral palsied child. She never walked or talked but she filled our home, and changed us from a couple to a family.

Too frequently, we hear that individuals so handicapped have no value, and perform no service. This just isn't true. Through her handicap her parents became interested in the problems of the mentally retarded and they took an active part in the creation of the local council for the retarded. This activity led to the establishment of other councils throughout the State of Indiana, and ultimately the creation of the Logan School locally, and other facilities and programs for the retarded elsewhere.

Yes, all this would have probably happened anyhow, but maybe not until a generation later.

And so Rita Jo, you did in your way serve humanity to the best of your ability, and with accomplishments much more evident than those of many persons much more favorably endowed in mind and body. And you served your parents too, for you taught them love and understanding; and though others may have thought you were our burden, actually you were our motivation, our spirit. Whatever we are today, we are better because you lived, and oh so thankful that you were ours.

---

A Mother's Thoughts

by Sophie Newman

1966

The most wonderful possession my husband and I ever had was a little girl named Rita Jo.

I always felt "God" sent me one of his angels by mistake, but decided if we were worthy enough He would leave her with us for a while. I did not know how long I could keep her, but I and my husband did everything we could possibly do to keep her stay on earth pleasant and fulfilling. We never regretted even one day of the 28 years that she lived. Each day was bright, and only when she was sick were we sad. We knew someday God would want her back, but we always hoped that would be in the far future. Our only wish was that she leave before we did, and the way to go was to just close your eyes and that was it. She went just that way. I was there and saw it all but never even realized she left this earth to go back to God. I was bathing her and making her comfortable at the time.

I am sure if there is such a "God" as I believe, He is very happy. She was precious on earth, and will be likewise in heaven. Many people believe that keeping and caring for such a child at home is a great mistake. This is not true. We had the privilege that comes to few people, that of having an angel in our own home. She molded our characters to her way as though they were made of clay. She gave us a great insight, and a compassion for others less fortunate than ourselves and an opportunity to make an effort to do something about it. Last but not least, she gave us great strength to be able to bear up to any pressure that might come our way in life, even her death and the loss that we feel so greatly. We realize that she is better off, and can now help us better than before because she has no crippled body to keep her back. We know she will never have a pain, and that what pain we have in losing her can be dulled by the thought that she will never have a day to suffer, that she is safe in the place all of us would wish to go to some day. "God" has given us great strength to bear our loss, because I am sure He feels we have done an excellent job of caring for one of his most cherished angels. We have the strength to bear our loss because she gave us the strength during her presence.

chapter 2

# The Right
# to Learn

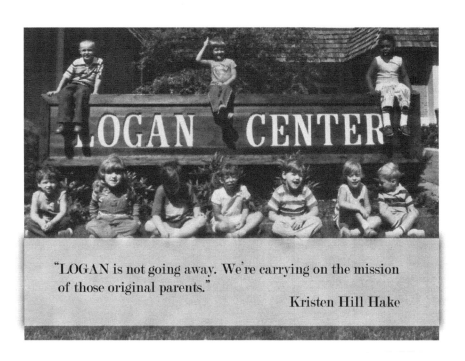

"LOGAN is not going away. We're carrying on the mission of those original parents."

Kristen Hill Hake

Competitors for some $900,000 in government grant money to assist citizens with disabilities had gathered to make their case before a health facilities council of about 30 people in Indianapolis in 1966. Methodist Hospital, which planned to devote an entire floor to mental health services, was the odds-on favorite.

Joe Doyle, president of the Council for the Retarded board, rose to make an impassioned plea for channeling the money to LOGAN School. Doyle, a prominent sports columnist for the *South Bend Tribune* covering Notre Dame football, had been trained in public speaking by Moose Krause, athletic director for the university, with one fundamental rule: "Talk until you think of something to say."

The building, old when LOGAN School started in 1950, was dangerously dilapidated, he said. Handicapped children, some on crutches, spent much of the day in the basement, a perilous firetrap. In fact, the Mishawaka fire marshal had threatened to shut down the operation entirely. Without the grant, these children would be out on the street, and the brave project launched by caring parents would collapse.

Leaving the meeting, LOGAN's Executive Director Mike Birkey turned to Doyle in horror: When had the fire marshal made such a threat? Birkey had never heard of it. What would they do if such a thing happened?

Well, the fire marshal hadn't really threatened, hadn't even really visited, Doyle confessed: "I built it up a little bit. But he could have been there. He could have done that. Come to think of it, he should have!"

Back in the committee, the vote went for Methodist Hospital, as expected. But as members gathered up their papers after the long day, a gentleman from downstate made a last-minute motion: If for some reason the Methodists turned down the government money, give the money to "that poor gentleman in South Bend to get the fire marshal off his back."

Motion passed. Methodist Hospital, after all, declined the state entanglement, freeing the money to build LOGAN Center.

"The fact that we got to build a building of our own was a good thing," said Doyle, who credits the high profile location on Eddy Street—across from the Notre Dame campus—with raising awareness.

Education was clearly LOGAN's first focus. LOGAN School, opened in 1950, was the fledgling group's first public face. The new building which opened in 1968 carried the name and the mission from Logan Street. Resembling more of a traditional school, the new LOGAN Center was a source of great pride to parents. The first maintenance director Vernon Batten, a World War II veteran, took the care of the new facility to heart. His son Denny was one of LOGAN's first students.

LOGAN's success at both providing services, such as those in the school building, and promoting advocacy, such as a state law that made education for students with disabilities a public responsibility, worked out well for both the students and the community.

By that time, advocacy success was overtaking service provision—the national movement for people with disabilities was winning rights to education that the Supreme Court ruled for African-Americans in 1954.

John Brademas, the local congressman and chair of the House Select Subcommittee on Education, was coauthor of the 1975 Education for All Handicapped Children Act. When an opponent on the floor of the House questioned spending resources on children who might learn no more than to put on their pants, Brademas retorted: "I don't know about you, Congressman, but it's awfully important to my success in life that I learned to put my pants on."

The State of Indiana passed a law in 1973 that required public school systems to provide education for all children, regardless of disability. In the mid-'70s, as the deadline approached for the mandate for special education, the South Bend Community School Corporation was pressured to provide that education—a service that LOGAN had been providing for some 20 years.

LOGAN leaders struck a deal with the schools: Classes could continue in the LOGAN Center on Eddy Street for three more years with corporation funding. After that, the schools would have to find their own space. With the state taking responsibility for special education, LOGAN shifted its focus to early childhood and adult services. Once the move was made by the school system, those LOGAN services, scattered in churches and other community space, would find their home at LOGAN Center.

The school corporation moved out of LOGAN Center in 1979 to classrooms in various buildings that segregated children with disabilities from the other students—the initial model for providing special education.

Kristen Hill Hake, who has a son with autism, remembers those days when people with disabilities were in separate classrooms, showing up at lunchtime and recess to be gawked at by the others. Now these students are fully integrated in the schools and enjoy pool parties and birthday parties with the rest of their class.

"Years ago, as a student myself, I was afraid of those kids with developmental disabilities," she recalled. "It's a different world now, and it's great. There's a lot of potential there. We have to embrace that and nurture that and realize that everybody has worth."

LOGAN connections long have championed full integration of students with disabilities in education. Pam von Rahl, past chair of LOGAN's Corporate Board and longtime director of Joint Services for Special Education for School City of Mishawaka/Penn-Harris-Madison School Corporation, led the movement far ahead of most of Indiana in the mid-1990s, insisting that the districts incorporate the children in neighborhood schools instead of self-contained buildings. She started with students with the most significant disabilities who had been sent to South Bend schools for services.

"People thought I'd lost my mind," she said, but the fruit of her approach has won broad acceptance. "It's not even controversial. Now it's the culture."

The central issue, von Rahl said, involves the impact of culture on individuals—students with disabilities, other students, special education teachers, and other teachers. In self-contained buildings, teachers who see only students with disabilities assume they will never learn to read. Teachers who labeled themselves "special education" had to break out of those roles and learn to problem-solve every day. "I watched special ed for years trying to simulate reality," she said.

Von Rahl said the first student moved into the mainstream achieved a yearlong Individual Education Plan (IEP) in less than three months in the new environment, surrounded by examples of ordinary language and behavior. Program assistants who work with the students support the inclusion. The students leave the room for certain activities when appropriate, but they maintain their dignity and identification with the class. "It is about membership," von Rahl said. "Where is my home? It's in third grade. Nice, segregated homes don't cut it. People look different when they have been integrated their whole life."

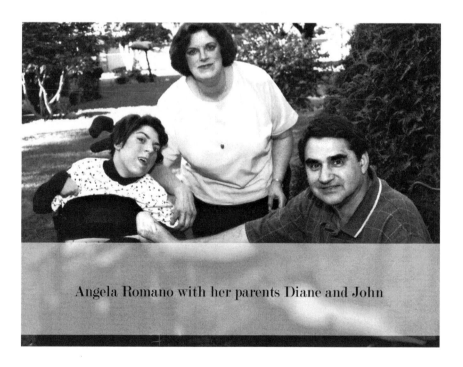

Angela Romano with her parents Diane and John

Students without disabilities quickly embraced their new classmates, she said: "They were like, 'OK, fine. Can I eat lunch with them? Can I push the wheelchair?' They get some sense that there is somebody different from me. Friendships are formed clear from kindergarten. We offer a class on peer mentoring." They also take their matter-of-fact interactions with those classmates home with them, spreading the fruit of inclusion to their families.

Diane Romano, a LOGAN activist whose daughter Angela attended South Bend's Clay High School, was head of a parent group for the school district when parents sued Indiana so students with special needs could continue to get educational programs to age 22, instead of age 18. The parents won.

"We brought these students back into the educational system," said Romano, who helped design a program to prepare the young adults for transition to vocational rehabilitation, setting a model for other districts in the state.

Achieving the goal of educational integration meant profound changes for an agency that had opened as a special school. A vast array of other services had already developed, including employment at LOGAN Industries, an adult rehabilitation program for individuals with severe disabilities, and a HomeStart Program started in 1970 for children from birth to age 5. In 1991, federal law mandated preschool for children ages 3 to 5 with special needs, something that LOGAN had offered for years even when other communities across the state had no such program. Indiana chose to meet this mandate by moving funding for the preschool program into the public schools, and, with this shift, the HomeStart program at LOGAN changed. LOGAN's early childhood program became Building Blocks for infants to 3-year-olds.

For three decades, families with school-age children with disabilities had no natural direct link to LOGAN—even if they received early services and expected to re-enter when the children reached age 22. As the 60th anniversary approached, LOGAN was expanding its community-service infrastructure to engage those people.

"Schools can't do everything for families," von Rahl said. "I'm pushing for LOGAN to offer more school-age services. LOGAN has always been in the community, supporting the dignity and purposeful life for these people."

## The Cleary Family

When Jo and Dick Cleary realized their son Dickie, at age 5 in 1963, was not developing normally, they quickly turned to the group of parents—LOGAN— that already had more than a decade of experience helping families deal with such issues.

As the next son and the next showed up with similar symptoms, eventually diagnosed as the progressive degenerative Hunter's syndrome, LOGAN stayed with the Clearys.

When the last son died at age 19, the Clearys stayed with LOGAN.

Dick, a University of Notre Dame graduate who managed a stock broker firm, never missed a meeting in 30 years on the LOGAN board. His participation with the National Center for Law and the Handicapped, housed at LOGAN Center, resulted in five national cases that won more rights for people with disabilities.

At one point, Dick got a significant promotion with his firm and the family moved to a posh Detroit suburb, but when the city's services failed to reach LOGAN standards, they came back in less than two years.

"We lived out in a nice, elegant part of Detroit," Jo says. "The problem was they didn't know anything about handicapped kids. They weren't educated as far as the handicapped in Detroit."

The Clearys first noticed an odd gait develop in Dickie's walking, and long-baffled doctors spent years performing tests and trying to diagnose the problem. Michael, two years younger, was not blind like the other two. Patrick, born in 1963, lived the longest, dying at age 19.

Jo happened to have started lifting weights when she was 25, so she was able to carry the boys as required.

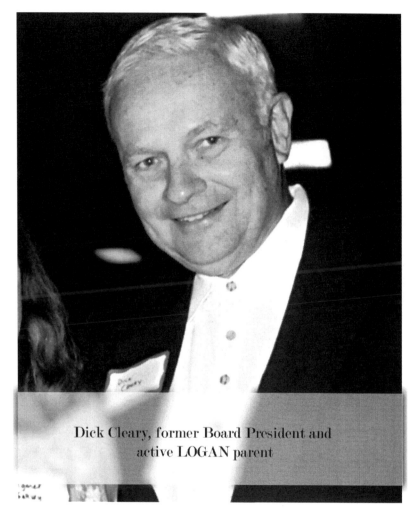

**Dick Cleary, former Board President and
active LOGAN parent**

"My first son weighed 50 pounds and I had to carry him up and down the stairs, and we had a quad level," Jo recalled. "The boys came first in every way, shape, or form."

The couple embraced the children as an identity-defining part of their life, like their Catholic faith and their love for Ireland and the Notre Dame Fighting Irish.

"That's what made us the way we were," Jo says. "We took it the way it was. This happened. All we could do was make them comfortable. Dick was an unusual person, and I was too, kind of. Even though crisis would come, there's always a way around it. I always had an upbeat attitude."

Their older (and only) daughter Colleen's fiancé was so impressed by the family's sacrifices and love for their sons that when they wed he changed his name to Cleary to carry the name forward.

LOGAN School was a key support for the family, with devoted teacher Mike Snyder regularly checking on the boys even when they weren't in his classroom. Jo volunteered frequently: "I would go over there during the day, and anything they wanted me to do, I would do." While Jo found her place at LOGAN in the classroom, Dick discovered his in the board room. The Clearys remained devoted to LOGAN for years after the deaths of their three sons.

## Joe Doyle

A year or two after LOGAN School opened, Joe Doyle's bartender-friend Lee Slaughter, an avid supporter of any children's program, volunteered him to help with something at the old building.

A couple of years later in 1957, Doyle had a daughter who was eventually diagnosed with profound mental retardation. She participated in LOGAN programs, until she moved into an institution in 1960. Doyle stayed involved, growing more and more active in the LOGAN group.

After he succeeded Dick Gamble as Council for the Retarded board president in 1963, Doyle held the position until 1969, maintaining necessary continuity through the years that the council was getting LOGAN Center built on Eddy Street.

"When I became president of LOGAN, I alienated half the mothers here," he said. "I said, 'This place is not going to run on bake sales.'"

Doyle, a *South Bend Tribune* columnist covering Notre Dame football since 1949, recruited his Air Force buddy, Erv Derda, to bring high-level business acumen to the organization.

With Derda's help, Joe turned to grants, United Way, county government, and his considerable connections to civic leaders and politicians for money to help pay for programs.

State property tax rules allowed up to two pennies on the tax rate to go to mental retardation work. The Council for the Retarded was getting one cent. When the county council president, a buddy of Doyle's, pointed out that no one had asked for the additional cent, the agency got some of that money, too.

Joe Newman and Joe Doyle at the
LOGAN Center groundbreaking, 1968

"The parents didn't just care about their own children. They cared about everyone's children — future children. That has always been the strength behind LOGAN."

Dan Harshman

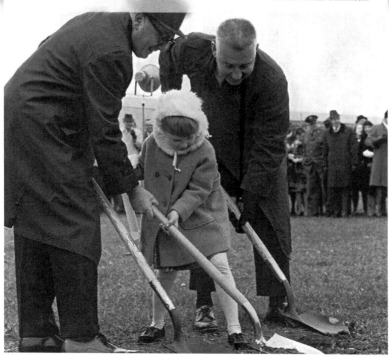

Early Thanksgiving morning of 1966, Rep. John Brademas called Doyle, asking him to come over to his house for a lobbying push to win Congressional appropriation for a grant to build the new LOGAN Center.

When Doyle, who was also preparing for a trip to California to cover the Notre Dame-USC game arrived, Brademas was on the phone with House Speaker John McCormack of Massachusetts. When that conversation ended, Brademas quickly called two more representatives before Doyle reminded him that it was a holiday morning.

"That's how they'll know it's important," Brademas explained. Notre Dame defeated USC 51-0 on Saturday. The appropriation passed Congress on Monday.

Doyle saw the importance of working the advocacy and services side of things simultaneously in order to strengthen both efforts.

"We were spending our time to build a building for the kids, while at the same time we were working with the legislature to get special education in the public schools," Doyle says. "We were working both sides. It worked out well because in the early days the schools used our building to teach their kids."

LOGAN bought land for the school from the state of Indiana, with Doyle and Dr. Stuart Ginsberg, chair of the health facilities council, exchanging the deed and a check for a few thousand dollars at a banquet one spring evening—the night Doyle was named St. Joseph Valley Notre Dame Alumni Club Man of the Year. Later that winter, with no record of either document on file, Doyle discovered the deed in his suit pocket and Ginsberg discovered the check in his coat pocket.

During construction, Doyle sometimes had to meet the state auditor to pick up the check needed to pay the contractor's installments on the $1.6 million project. Once when payments were due, Doyle got a $300,000 loan from First State Bank on his signature, and bank officials assured examiners that United Way had backed the transaction with a verbal agreement.

Negotiations over how to heat the building—electricity, gas, or power from the neighboring Northern Indiana Children's Hospital—led to a contract with the electric company. A tape recording of the meetings saved thousands of dollars when the utility company attempted to charge more than agreed.

After LOGAN Center was built, Doyle wanted to hire a doctor to run a diagnostic clinic in the building, but the agency's application for a federal grant was rejected.

On a side trip to Washington from a Notre Dame-Navy game, Doyle and a half-dozen other LOGAN leaders appealed to government health officials to reconsider, but they met stony silence.

Doyle, angry, strode ahead of the others as they left down a long hall, until he happened to notice the exact dollar amount of the grant scribbled on a blackboard in one of the rooms—along with a half-dozen criteria for the award.

He quietly copied the criteria, rewrote the grant along those lines when he returned to South Bend, and got a call within the week that the money had been awarded. The clinic operated from the late 1960s to the late 1970s.

## The Hay Family

Just two weeks from giving birth to her second child, Bonnie Hay was volunteering at the 1987 International Special Olympics in South Bend when she happened to have a conversation with the mother of an Olympian with Down syndrome.

"She was telling me that her son was always happy to see her when she got home, always asked about her day and was always concerned," Bonnie recalled. "I thought, 'How bad can this be?'"

She remembered those words when Dr. Robert White told Bonnie and Brian that their newborn daughter, Stephanie, had mosaic Down syndrome, a milder-than-usual but still shocking turn for the family whose son Connor was just a toddler.

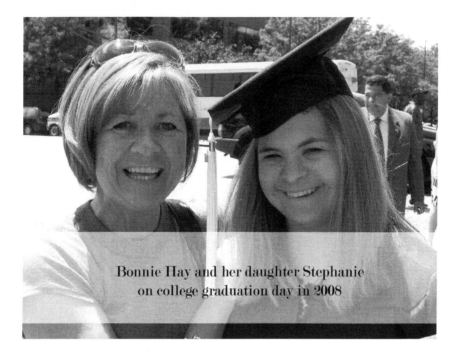

**Bonnie Hay and her daughter Stephanie
on college graduation day in 2008**

"We can do this," said the couple, who had earlier lost a set of twins. "We already know and love her."

They also knew LOGAN would help. Bonnie had grown up volunteering with her parents at the agency's huge Christmas party at LOGAN Center where her brother-in-law played Santa, and the LOGAN clients always won the basketball game.

Stephanie received therapies and preschool services through LOGAN's HomeStart program, and the family decided to send her to St. Anthony School despite its lack of services for students with special needs.

"The principal embraced the idea and set the tone for everyone," Bonnie recalls. "She wanted her teachers to learn from Stephanie so that they could become better teachers."

By the time Stephanie finished the eighth grade, she was reading to younger students and helping them with spelling and journaling.

"It's not what the community does for these kids—there's a whole reciprocation that doesn't get acknowledged," Bonnie says. "That's what St. Anthony's School did. By allowing that reciprocation to happen, they learned so much from Stephanie."

Meanwhile, Stephanie was participating in the family ski trips and a camp in Colorado where she landed a job helping with the horses and leading trail songs for the riders.

Stephanie finished high school with the help of her teacher of record, Bonnie Miller, and went on to National Lewis University in Chicago for a program designed for students with learning challenges. To encourage other students and their families, Stephanie gave a PowerPoint presentation of her college experience at LOGAN's first College Fair, an event initially prompted by families with children on the autism spectrum but expanded to options for students with all learning challenges.

Advice that Bonnie received when Stephanie was a baby helped her keep focus for years.

"Another mom of a child with special needs once told me not to be so concerned with 5 or 10 years down the road, because you won't be able to enjoy the moment," she recalls. "We took that advice to heart and learned to let Stephanie guide us. After all, it is her life."

chapter 3

# Real Jobs

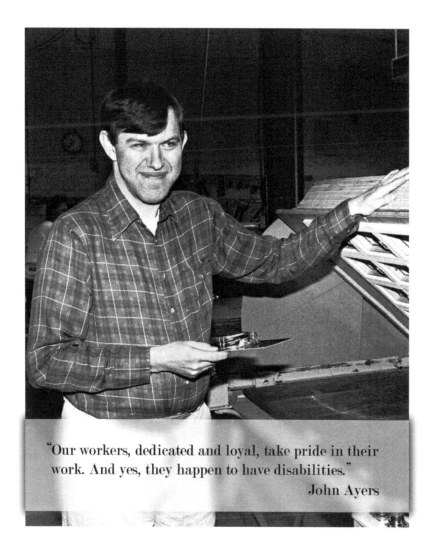

"Our workers, dedicated and loyal, take pride in their work. And yes, they happen to have disabilities."

John Ayers

A s a financial officer at Clark Equipment Co., Erv Derda knew how a modern business ought to operate. As a member of the LOGAN board, he wanted LOGAN Industries to operate that way. So Derda optioned a parcel of land in the developing industrial park near the South Bend Airport with $10,000 of his own money. Newly-hired LOGAN Chief Executive Officer Dan Harshman, approaching legislators for the first of many times during his career, secured a state grant for $2.7 million—the largest of its kind at the time. Jim Gibbons, a LOGAN board member who had been involved with the local Special Olympics, enlisted his colleague Jim Frick, Notre Dame's vice president of Public Relations, and the high-powered leaders quickly raised the remaining cash necessary to build a 90,000-square-foot facility for the sheltered workshop. Workers moved into the new building in 1981, a far cry from the dilapidated building on High Street that had been LOGAN's employment center for more than a decade.

"I was used to modern manufacturing and administrative facilities. I felt we should build a building," Derda recalled. "LOGAN parents thought I had lost my mind. Little by little, we got the community involved. We leaned on our business contacts to start talking to people. What I felt was important was to build a modern manufacturing facility which could then compete for work and run it as a business. LOGAN Industries was set up as a not-for-profit, but that didn't mean for a loss."

The industrial park location was strategic not only for exposure to potential customers but also for the larger LOGAN vision of full community integration. "Other people would see our folks coming to work, riding the bus, waiting for the bus to go home," Derda said.

35

Employment had been part of LOGAN's mission nearly from the beginning, with initiatives launched just five years after the school opened. From the very start, the comprehensive approach included both community-based jobs and workshop jobs that were conducted at various locations around town. As it expanded, LOGAN Industries moved from a 17,000-square-foot former automobile dealership in downtown Mishawaka to the 59,000-square-foot former South Bend Tackle Shop near downtown South Bend in 1966, before settling in its new 90,000-square-foot manufacturing facility in the industrial park. Even as the workshop grew, LOGAN sustained its focus on both workshop and community-based jobs.

The Employment Services Program, aimed at local businesses who would hire LOGAN clients, started in 1986. LOGAN provided training and follow-up for the workers, who approached their jobs with eager diligence.

"We were always looking for employers that were open and flexible, people who were tolerant and patient with an optimistic point of view," recalled Sue Correa, who was working in community employment placement 20 years ago. One of the first placements came at Martin's Super Markets, a community-minded company that went on to hire several other workers with disabilities. The first man hired, a bagger, received a new bicycle from the store on his 10th anniversary. Another worker with Down syndrome, a favorite of loyal grocery shoppers, earned a special recognition badge to wear on his uniform.

In 1988, Correa was trying to place several young men who had finished high school with minimal job skills. Seeking more options for employment, she called a car dealership where she reached an unusually receptive employer.

"This sales guy was wonderful—he was optimistic, upbeat, and listened to our speech about employees with support," Correa recalled. "He said, 'I just need to know they are willing to work and have an interest in employment.' He told me that he had had some challenging years when he was younger."

The dealership hired one of the men as a go-between in the body shop. The salesman turned out to be Rudy Ruettiger, the University of Notre Dame football walk-on whose story became a popular movie. The employees of the Gurley Leep Automotive Family welcomed Trent Paluchniak, who worked at the dealership for years and always somehow won the cash prize at the staff holiday party. Trent's work drew Mike Leep, Sr., the dealership's owner, into the LOGAN mission as a board member, and he became a leading donor and community advocate.

Perhaps the most challenging placement ever accomplished involved Jeannie Bunyon, who lived at a nursing home and had no use of her muscles. She typed on a computer by blowing through a straw—three words per minute. A manufacturing company hired her to transcribe meeting notes with adapted equipment. Volunteers from Notre Dame and Saint Mary's College, inspired by her determination, helped whenever needed with such tasks as feeding paper into a printer.

In the early 1990s, LOGAN opened two affirmative businesses, Boland Quality Manufacturing and LOGAN Contract Services, to increase employment opportunities. These businesses eventually closed as attention turned more to other companies for hiring. Other agencies started providing more support for community-based work. In 2006, LOGAN decided to concentrate on LOGAN Industries while encouraging individuals to work part-time in the community and part-time at the workshop. Workers who could not find full-time employment in the community could get flexible hours at LOGAN Industries, and those who had community jobs could stay connected with the workshop.

"Unfortunately, the community is not able to employ everyone," said Rob Palmer, LOGAN's CFO who oversees the work center. "I think workshops are a viable alternative to that. There are a lot of great companies out there that do employ persons with disabilities, but many of them are underemployed. Some people hold jobs both at LOGAN Industries and outside companies, where they might work only two days a week. They'll come in and work the other three days at the workshop. They want full employment."

As the 60th anniversary of LOGAN approached, in the midst of the deepest economic downturn in its history, the workshop employed over 160 people and was enjoying its busiest time. Some entrepreneurial businesses that started with LOGAN had grown rapidly, and LOGAN Industries added a second salesperson. At the same time, a few companies that suffered layoffs found themselves with more business and turning to LOGAN rather than prematurely recalling employees. LOGAN workers, paid by the piece, got a chance to practice increased productivity.

"We train our workers and try to keep them very busy. There's definitely the social aspect of being around their friends—just like any other type of job," Palmer said. "We run it like a business because it gives them what would be expected if they went out and were employed in the community, such as showing up on time, getting back from lunch on time, staying on task. There are a lot of things that can position them for community employment. That's their job. It's not just a place to go."

"I still think people don't understand what we're doing at LOGAN Industries," said John Ayers, sales manager for 33 years. "Most have no idea of the span of services we offer and the equipment we utilize." A revamp of the website geared to manufacturers, which for years did not mention that the workers were people with disabilities, now integrates such information about the workforce along with an emphasis on quality. "We don't lead with that card, but we don't hide that card. Our workers, dedicated and loyal, take pride in their work. And yes, they happen to have disabilities."

Much of the work involves packaging, assembly, or tagging, with products from sockets to cat food treats to Pinewood Derby kits. Some workers use aids such as a template that shows four wheels and four nails for the worker to gather and package in a labeled tube. Workers quickly pick up the routine and are able to repeat it accurately. "We're no different from any other facility," Palmer said. "We have a lot of quality control, a lot of quality checks. We have long-established customers. They depend on us and we depend on them. When customers find a mistake, we're just like any other company—send it back and we'll fix it. We have to be competitive in the marketplace. There are independent packaging companies out there. We're out there quoting jobs just like anybody else."

A consortium of similar workshops across Indiana formed in 2004, with leaders meeting quarterly to share experiences, study best practices, hear legislative updates from state officials, tour each others' facilities, and sometimes develop collaborations. The group started with representatives from six work centers and within five years had grown to 20 workshops represented, including operations in Elkhart, Valparaiso, and Michigan City and as far south as Indianapolis and Columbus.

In an effort to integrate workers with developmental disabilities into the larger workforce, Michigan closed its workshops. But LOGAN leaders maintained that a continuum of opportunities best serves the workers. Community employment is scarce—often limiting workers to 16 hours a week with little long-term security—especially in a recessionary climate with high unemployment. Workshops like LOGAN Industries are valued by workers and their families because they provide an important social and educational setting as well as jobs.

Customers also value the workshops. Chuck Kelderhouse, owner of Georgia-based KAHOOT Products that produces the famous Boy Scout Pinewood Derby kits, depends on LOGAN Industries for packaging. "Our relationship with LOGAN Industries has been long term," he said. "They have always given us the confidence that we could grow our product line while meeting our customer demands."

LOGAN Industries' customer mix ranges from small local businesses to large corporations, such as Whirlpool and AM General. Customers initially attracted to LOGAN Industries for the range of services may not realize at first the unique workforce. Impressed by the quality of services delivered, they gain respect for the skills and dedication of the workers and gain satisfaction for their own role in offering such employment opportunities.

# Erv Derda

Erv Derda became a LOGAN parent more than 40 years after he joined LOGAN's board of directors. But his work for people with disabilities was always personal.

Erv, a World War II Air Force pilot, was financial officer at Clark Equipment when his flying buddy Joe Doyle asked him to bring his business expertise to the parent group that was mostly holding bake sales to meet its budget. He joined the board later in 1957 and served as president from 1970 -1973. His personal and business connections have benefited people with disabilities for decades.

In addition to his LOGAN service, Erv joined the President's Commission on Mental Retardation in the Carter administration and channeled money to the National Center for Law and the Handicapped, a joint venture between LOGAN and the University of Notre Dame, housed at LOGAN Center, where he was on the board from 1980 to 1988. He was also a member of the Indiana Association for Retarded Citizens board.

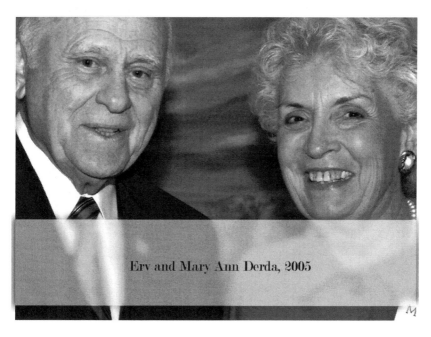

Erv and Mary Ann Derda, 2005

Under Erv's direction, LOGAN built a $4 million, 90,000-square-foot manufacturing facility for LOGAN Industries near the South Bend airport, replacing a run-down facility on High Street where workshop activities had been consolidated in 1969.

He led the organization of the 1987 International Special Olympics held at the University of Notre Dame, a project six years in the making, with the support of his wife Irene and his employer. Erv retired from Clark Equipment in 1986 in order to devote full time to the last year of preparations. He became president of the LOGAN Foundation, launched with profits from the Special Olympics, but wrote a two-year term limit into the bylaws in order to hand off the responsibility.

Erv's son Jeff became president of the board for Camp Millhouse, a facility for people with disabilities, and his daughter Susan writes briefs for justices at the Division of Special Education in New York. Irene died in 2002.

In 2003, he married Mary Ann Matthews, whose husband Dave died in 1990, and took the role of father to her son Kevin, who has a disability. Over the years, their paths had crossed many times at LOGAN. Mary Ann was on LOGAN's board in 1968, when Erv was president, and a member of the Camp Millhouse board when Jeff was president.

Erv perceives his social responsibility to people with disabilities as seriously as he takes his new personal responsibilities for Kevin, who gets Air Force-style discipline on policing his room balanced by a monthly guys' night out with his stepfather. Jeff always joked about Erv's "non-parent" designation among LOGAN folks, wondering where that placed him in the equation. At last, Erv officially earned his spot as a LOGAN parent. But for decades, Erv was an example that the parents of people with disabilities are not alone in the responsibility for the well-being of their children—we all are. Some of us accept this direct role on behalf of all of us.

Erv taught Kevin, who has worked at LOGAN Industries since 1985, how to respond to some people who suggest that his LOGAN Industries work isn't a "real" job: "I ask him, 'When you go to the bank and cash your check, do they give you real money?'"

chapter **4**

# An Awakened
# Conscience

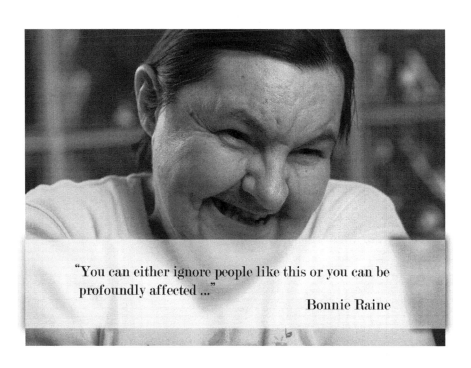

"You can either ignore people like this or you can be profoundly affected ..."

Bonnie Raine

W hen a resident of Riverside Center suffered gross abuse at the hands of a facility employee, St. Joseph County Prosecutor Michael Barnes sent a police officer as an undercover agent to investigate conditions at the institution overlooking the St. Joseph River next to Indiana University South Bend. The victim was a ward of LOGAN's guardianship program. The agent, hired as an aide, uncovered large-scale neglect and abuse of dozens of residents with developmental disabilities, most of them in their 20s. The episode revealed a hitherto-overlooked consequence of well-intentioned government policies, a suffering population, and the ill-equipped staff assigned to serve them, and the call for a host of support services to provide a life of safety and dignity for forgotten human beings.

LOGAN's involvement in the episode confirmed its original, undivided commitment to both advocacy and service, providing a clear voice for the voiceless as well as a helping hand for the helpless. The agency's Protective Services took on a role unimagined and far broader than expected when it formed to care for LOGAN's own clients after their parents were gone. But the expanded role was the inevitable result of LOGAN's unwavering commitment to its mission.

Since the mid-1970s, Riverside had taken in people with disabilities to keep its beds filled. Indiana, like other states, was de-institutionalizing individuals with severe disabilities in recognition of their rights as human beings. But the state did not provide sufficient resources or planning for an effective transition into society, and many who left state institutions wound up in nursing homes and other private institutions like Riverside.

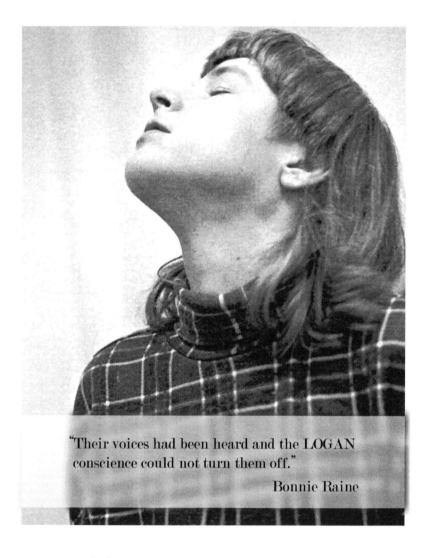

"Their voices had been heard and the LOGAN conscience could not turn them off."

Bonnie Raine

One particularly strong advocate was a father whose son lived at NISH (Northern Indiana State Hospital), formerly known as the Northern Indiana Children's Hospital. He was concerned about former residents who had been moved to Riverside when they became adults. He alerted LOGAN to the concentration of need in the facility, and LOGAN workers began to offer programming under its Adult Rehabilitation Program, which later became Adult Day Services. This was the first time LOGAN had provided such programming for individuals with very significant disabilities. Most of the Riverside residents were nonverbal with extreme physical challenges, living much of their lives in bed or in hard plastic institutional chairs.

The LOGAN staff sensed something amiss in the environment, but their limited contact failed to uncover the depth of trouble until the Blizzard of 1978. With the Riverside staff unable to reach the residents due to the 30 inches of snow that had fallen, LOGAN Protective Services staff and volunteers organized to provide continuous care and feeding—and the institution's shortcomings could no longer remain hidden.

"This was the first time that LOGAN had spent extended time in this facility, but it wasn't the last," recalled Bonnie Raine, director of LOGAN's Protective Services staff. "What they experienced firsthand was neglect and substandard conditions, things that these residents had endured for years. LOGAN began to get more involved, spending more time at Riverside. Now, knowing what we knew about the conditions that these people endured, there was no turning back. Their voices had been heard and the LOGAN conscience could not turn them off."

The company had left the residents' care to low-wage workers unaware of their needs and unable to care for them. They were left in fetal positions, their weight dropping to 80 to 100 pounds, their bodies deformed with muscular-skeletal abnormalities developed from long inactivity.

Alerted to the issues by LOGAN, the owners tried to improve conditions. The business hired a rehabilitation company for speech, occupational, and physical therapy. It bought expensive plastic molded scoop chairs so patients could get out of bed, unaware that the one size would not fit the bodies of individuals with very different physical disabilities. LOGAN's Adult Rehabilitation staff, unable to provide adequate services in the environment, withdrew, but Protective Services kept watch, sending a team led by Dr. Dick Reineke, a LOGAN parent, to assess the individuals so that LOGAN could prepare to better support them.

By 1980, concerned for the residents' safety, LOGAN convinced Michael Barnes, the prosecutor, to investigate the institution. When the undercover effort exposed the conditions, Barnes charged the owners with four counts of neglect of a dependent adult. A judge turned down an attempt by Riverside's lawyers to block LOGAN from moving the residents. LOGAN clearly needed to take guardianship in order to gain control of the situation. Barnes worked with LOGAN to take corporate guardianship of 27 individuals in one day, after efforts to engage their families failed.

On Halloween night of 1981, a crew of LOGAN staff and volunteers, including Dan Harshman and Bonnie Raine, arrived at the building like so many storm troopers with a fleet of specialized wheelchair-carrying vans. They quickly gathered the residents' belongings and relocated them all overnight to another nursing facility across town. The facility was closed.

Nobody was thinking of Riverside residents when LOGAN started its Protective Services Board for advocacy and guardianship services in 1974. Most of the members were thinking of themselves and their own children.

The love of a parent for a disabled child has two conflicting consequences: a natural desire for the child to live and an understandable fear for the child that outlives parents and must go on without their care. Variations of that struggle, sometimes involving siblings and other relatives, can tear at the fabric of relationships. Among other things, having a child with a disability statistically increases the likelihood of divorce.

Some parents pray every day that their child will die before they do. Some resist that mindset. When one LOGAN parent's devout relative mentioned that she prays every day "that the Lord will take your daughter," the mother retorted: "I'm afraid that we're praying at cross purposes."

From the beginning of LOGAN, Joe Newman argued that the agency should become a solution to that problem. No number of services, however wonderful, could suffice as long as the fundamental question of the future remained for individuals with disabilities and their families. A mother ought not to have to worry about outliving her daughter.

"It's a criticism of society," he said. "That mother is saying, 'I can't trust you to take care of my child. Parents are saying, 'I don't trust society.' "

LOGAN became the agent of society for looking after these children—not a substitute to relieve society of that responsibility, but a way for society to fulfill that role. Further, the Arc of Indiana has developed a trust option designed to help parents plan financially for their child's future.

Stanley Hauerwas, an ethicist at Notre Dame on the LOGAN Corporate Board of Directors in the late 1970s, was liaison between that board and the Protective Services Board. He trained the board, staff, and volunteers and drafted LOGAN's medical code policy before he left to become a professor at Duke University. His writings on moral dilemmas in the care of people with mental retardation sometimes reference cases from LOGAN. Touched by the South Bend group, Hauerwas dedicated his book *Suffering Presence* "to the people who comprise the Council for the Retarded of St. Joseph County, Ind."

"Having Stanley on the board was another example of LOGAN being visionary," said Bonnie Raine, whose doctoral dissertation Hauerwas directed. "LOGAN clearly wanted to stretch beyond itself and build a larger, more coherent context for its thinking, its commitment, and its work."

Only four years after Protective Services began on behalf of its clients and their families, the role carried LOGAN into the once-invisible world of Riverside and its ilk.

"We thought we'd be supporting these parents and their kids in school, when they got older," Dan Harshman said. "But then we found this terrible flaw in the system—all these people who had been abandoned into nursing homes. That got us into this other world of people who had been abandoned, the result of that whole institutionalization of 30 years before us. We were starting to see the underbelly of that. We only had one staff person in Protective Services, but we took this on."

It was, one hopes, the last generation of people deprived of education, services, and treatment appropriate to both their disabilities and their abilities. The movement started in the 1950s was bearing fruit for the rising generation, but for LOGAN, older people left helpless through no fault of their own had the same rights and value.

In the early 1970s, Indiana considered closing NISH, which shared the block with LOGAN.

"In a sense, Northern Indiana Children's Hospital should indeed be closed—as we have known this institution for the last decade," Linden Thorn, executive director of the Council for the Retarded, wrote to the local newspaper in 1972. "But its doors should remain open for the new kind of institution it can and should become. Simply to shut down Children's Hospital and scatter its unprepared occupants to whatever substitute care arrangement may be available would be a tragedy and the worst sort of misplaced 'economy.'"

The institution stayed open, but residents needed better living conditions and programming not available at the underfunded nursing care facility where broken windows had been boarded up for years. The children attended LOGAN Center for education daily.

"Until society rids itself of the institutionalization syndrome that only wastes financial resources and dehumanizes those it professes to serve and instead embraces and supports a concept that allows its retarded citizens to lead lives as normal as possible by providing educational and training programs designed to help them cope with the outside world, we will continue to be confronted with tragedies like NICH," Mike Snyder, a LOGAN School teacher wrote to the newspaper in 1972.

In the late 1970s, LOGAN even had to advocate against NISH. The hospital was in the habit of moving residents to nursing homes, where costs were a fraction of the hospital expenses. In a class action lawsuit against the state, a parent group won the right for children up to age 22 to stay at NISH for active programming and therapies made available in recent years.

LOGAN became the guardian or representative payee for people with severe disabilities and those whose disabilities fell short of thresholds for government programs but left them struggling with daily life for lack of a support system.

"You're deciding their groceries, their personal needs, their medical treatment, or the treatment they're getting where they live," Harshman said.

"It pushed us into a world most of our colleagues had not yet entered. They didn't know there was a problem in nursing homes. It wasn't on their plate either psychologically or in their budget. This commitment to those most vulnerable has been a unique thing to LOGAN, a real thread in our history. We knew we were sitting on a big systemic problem."

Once the LOGAN conscience awakened, there was no turning back, no choice but to take action. In 2004, LOGAN filed a class action lawsuit (*Kraus vs. Hamilton*) on behalf of an individual for whom LOGAN Protective Services took guardianship who was moved from one nursing home to another out of his community, because there was no other place for him to go. The lawsuit was not just on behalf of Tommy Kraus. It represented an estimated 1,800 such adults living in nursing homes in Indiana—the fourth highest rate nationwide, according to a 2008 report by David Braddock, Ph.D., and Richard Hemp, M.A., for the Indiana Institute on Disability and Community. The lawsuit called for the state of Indiana to provide more resources for community living options for people with developmental disabilities misplaced in nursing homes because of no alternatives. Further, the lawsuit directed the state of Indiana to inform these individuals of their rights to other housing, such as apartments or group homes. The problem persists. Many have known no life outside of institutions and are afraid to move. Efforts to inform these individuals continue, but in the first five years after the lawsuit, only 150 people have left nursing homes for community housing.

Looking back, the Riverside experience became a defining moment for LOGAN, sealing its commitment to all those with developmental disabilities, not just the ones with parents to advocate for them.

"One of the greatest things that came out of this crisis was that people made connections with others they may not have otherwise met," Harshman said. "This whole event and the circumstances leading up to it came to define what LOGAN was about. We reaffirmed a sense of responsibility for people who didn't have families.

"Some parents expressed concern about this new focus, worried whether LOGAN would remain attentive to their families. LOGAN responded by saying that parents need to help the organization help those who do not have families, because this is the strongest proof of the commitment that LOGAN will be there for their son or daughter when they are no longer there."

# Bonnie Raine

LOGAN Protective Services worker Bonnie Raine's heart leaped as soon as she saw an ABC television report on orphanages in Romania for children with disabilities.

"These are our folks!" she said, recognizing the common humanity and the common need half a world away.

Raine would know.

Mentored by Joe Newman and hired by the Council for the Retarded in 1978 to follow NISH graduates to their new institutional homes, the onetime Notre Dame theology graduate student had discovered the potential in such faces.

"LOGAN stepped up to the plate to defend the most vulnerable, helpless, and devalued people in our community," Raine said. "Devalued people need to have access to socially valued, culturally valued services of support. They disappear from the face of the earth and we get some subtle message that they are not as good, not as valuable as the rest of us."

There was James Paul, the young man at the Riverside Center nursing home with cerebral palsy, severe deformities, no ability to speak, and deep brown eyes that opened a wide window to his soul.

Once when Raine was alone with him, she started mocking the one-size-fits-all "spoon chairs" bought to bring residents with physical disabilities out of bed—and James Paul's twinkling eyes confirmed the meaning of his cackling laughter: "You got it, sister. You know exactly what I think about all of this." She enjoyed his engaging sense of humor and friendship until he died in the mid-1980s.

During the Blizzard of 1978, when Raine was among LOGAN workers caring for residents with developmental disabilities at River-

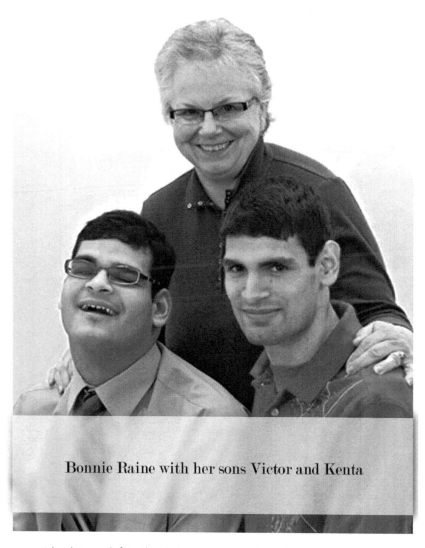

Bonnie Raine with her sons Victor and Kenta

side, she was left in the darkness one evening with a young woman who could not talk and who could move only by scooting with her one good leg.

"You can either ignore people like this or you can be profoundly affected, understanding that there is a greater presence and responsibility," she thought as she carried on a one-sided conversation with the woman. "No one would really know that I was here tonight except me, God, and you. Who would know? But I believe that you want me here."

When the news about Romanian orphans reached LOGAN, occupational therapist Jane Schmidt volunteered to go for a couple of visits, taking clothes, food, and toys; providing therapy; fashioning equipment; and bringing back stories about the children.

Jane's involvement further inspired Raine who started visiting and decided to adopt, overcoming the fear of Romanian officials that Americans seeking such adoptions might harvest organs for transplant.

Now, years later, she has two teenage sons with disabilities, continuing in a personal way the mission she carried out professionally at LOGAN.

"The heart of LOGAN is to say these people have value no matter where they are," Raine said. "Who in the next decade will LOGAN serve? What will be the next challenge? LOGAN will rise to that."

chapter 5

# Adding Quality
to Life

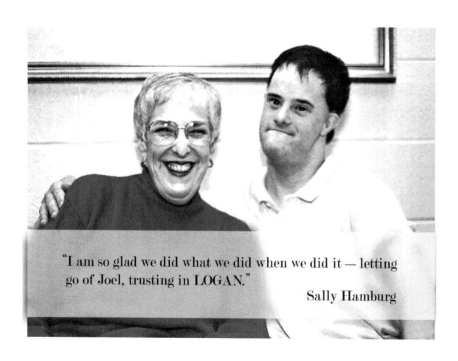

"I am so glad we did what we did when we did it — letting
go of Joel, trusting in LOGAN."

Sally Hamburg

The Riverside experience revealed not only the safety issues faced by people with disabilities but also their need for day-in, day-out experiences that affirm their dignity and worth. The need was especially acute in South Bend, partly because of NISH, LOGAN's neighbor across from campus, that brought an unusual number of children with severe disabilities from across Indiana to St. Joseph County.

As the children aged, and state policy moved away from such institutionalization, the need multiplied for services to people not suited for employment. At the same time, some LOGAN families' children with multiple disabilities were reaching adulthood. Although programming for these people was relatively new and not yet fully developed, LOGAN stepped up to start a program to meet the need to provide a better quality of life.

LOGAN's first class for adults with more significant disabilities opened at LOGAN Center on Eddy Street. Space limits in the building kept the program to one room, but other Adult Rehabilitation Program sites opened at NISH and nearby churches and nursing homes. At last, the onetime "lost generation"—too old for the education rights recently won for people with disabilities—was getting well-deserved attention through therapy and programming. The program became known as Adult Day Services, and a parent group formed that raised money for more supplies and services.

Many of the people turned out of institutions such as Riverside and the state hospital were not best suited for work at LOGAN Industries—some because their disabilities had been extreme from the beginning, some because they had grown up without the education and therapy that could have helped them. LOGAN organized to meet their needs.

"We reached out to them when there wasn't anything available for these people and developed a program for them at some risk financially," Dan Harshman said. "This got us into more comprehensive programming than the sheltered workshop. These are people who needed so much basic care."

The program started with 10 people in one classroom in 1978, but boosted with government funds (Title XX), it grew to nearly 100 people and demanded more space, part of the reason LOGAN insisted that the public schools leave the building on Eddy Street. Trends in the field moved away from facility-based programs to community-based programs—a false either-or, from LOGAN's point of view. "We think there's a place for both," Harshman emphasized. "Options should be comprehensive."

The original basic curriculum expanded to include music, art, gardening, exercise, cooking, and special events such as dances and parties. Specialized transportation made more community-based options available. Today, participants volunteer in such community activities as delivering Meals on Wheels, working at a food bank, cleaning up parks, recycling, shelving books at the library, and helping at churches. These activities make them real contributors, helping others in the community and gaining a sense of their own worth. The program includes community events and recreation activities such as Fridays at the Fountain, a popular South Bend lunchtime outdoor music event, as well as swimming and workouts at the YMCA.

Recreation became a vital part of life at LOGAN for many who did not have the skills or social supports and needed the program's structure. Bill Locke, the first recreation director, expanded offerings to include overnight camping, day camps, dances, parties, swimming, scouting, art and theater, and excursions to Chicago—mostly to cheer on the Cubs. LOGAN Center, once a school-day place, had become a hub of evening and weekend activity, and the community was getting used to seeing people with disabilities out and about. Among other things, students at Notre Dame donated their football tickets for the season-ending game. Exuberant LOGAN fans warmed the student section in November and attracted more volunteers to the center in an upward spiral of mutual support.

Person Centered Planning, an approach started at LOGAN years before it became a state initiative in the 1990s, brought more focus on the individual needs of the person, rather than fitting them into prepackaged services. Parents and professionals would meet with the individual to discern what they wanted most out of life. If the client could not articulate their opinions, a close friend would speak for them. This process tailored a mix of activities for individuals, such as working part-time at LOGAN Industries and volunteering at a local hospital.

As in the broader society, the aging population impacted LOGAN services. Many adults were entering their senior years, ready to retire from work at LOGAN Industries or wishing for a day program better suited to their needs. LOGAN's loyalty to these individuals, many of whom had been with the agency throughout their lives, led to the creation of a seniors program. Starting with a small group, the service has grown to include 46 people in several classrooms at the LOGAN Industries building. Games, favorite television shows, art, gardening, and social activities bring older friends together.

LOGAN has always served both ends of the age spectrum, although the movement of education into the public schools meant little contact with families of children that age. In recent years, the agency worked to restore a more continuous relationship by offering recreation and autism services to school-age families.

LOGAN's HomeStart Program launched in 1972 with a class of 10 active 2-year-olds. Therapists and developmental teachers also went into homes, working with infants and toddlers and teaching their caregivers ways to further the development of the child. This approach continues in LOGAN's early intervention program, now called Building Blocks. Parents of that original small group of preschoolers, including Sally Hamburg who had moved to South Bend with her son Joel in 1971, became close and organized ongoing gatherings and parties for the families.

HomeStart soon added a preschool program for children up to 5 in the LOGAN Center classrooms where students had previously attended school before public education took over that responsibility. The proximity to Notre Dame and Saint Mary's College brought numerous volunteers. Relationships developed during those critical early years made parents reluctant to part when their children entered public schools. HomeStart held a cap-and-gown graduation for the 5-year-olds in the gym, and they left LOGAN, usually not returning until they turned 18.

When the state shifted responsibility for education starting at age 3 to the schools, the change sharply reduced LOGAN's HomeStart program and opened space for more adult programs at the center. Building Blocks, as the program became known in 1994, continued, operating at a financial loss, yet LOGAN maintained the conviction that early intervention is vital to the children's well-being. The program added summer camps and sensory classes for older children.

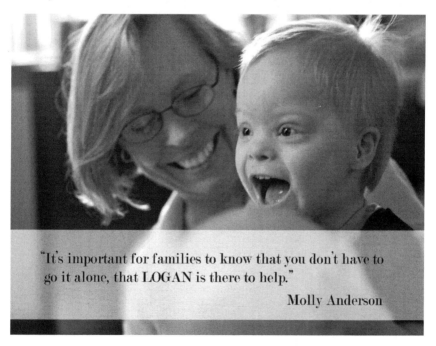

"It's important for families to know that you don't have to go it alone, that LOGAN is there to help."

Molly Anderson

In 2002, LOGAN created a Resource Center, a library of materials about disabilities and opportunities to provide information for families, not only about disabilities but also about camping options, wheelchair-friendly vacation spots, therapeutic horseback riding, new communication devices and therapy techniques, and dentists who offered services for children with autism or other sensory issues. LOGAN started a free Outreach Series for families and professionals covering such topics as Future Planning, Recreation Activities and Respite, Parenting, and Adapted Equipment.

The opening of the Regional Autism Center in 2004 once more connected LOGAN with school-age families. Down syndrome families, who had their own Michiana Down Syndrome Family and Advocacy Support Group, approached LOGAN about offering more for school-age children. The agency hired a recreation therapist in 2010 to develop more options to meet these needs. Activities included cooking, art, gardening, community trips, a teen group paired with Bethel College students, and a summer camp with the help of Notre Dame football players.

Looking back at the progression of her son's life with LOGAN, from toddler to adult, Sally Hamburg is struck by the expansion of services through the years as the organization stepped up to meet changing needs. Yet, she continually reminds LOGAN that the true measure of success is in the quality of the lives of those served. Keeping individuals, like her son Joel, at the very heart of services is imperative, she contends: "It's not a program, it's my son's life."

## The Anderson Family

Molly Lennon Anderson's father, Chuck Lennon, the director of the Alumni Association for the University of Notre Dame, was the legal guardian for a LOGAN client named Frankie while Molly was growing up. LOGAN was part of Lennon life. Chuck and his wife Joan chaperoned LOGAN dances and took Molly and their four other children with them to visit Frankie in the nursing home.

The lesson of LOGAN came home even more powerfully when Molly and her husband Kevin had their first child, KJ, so prematurely

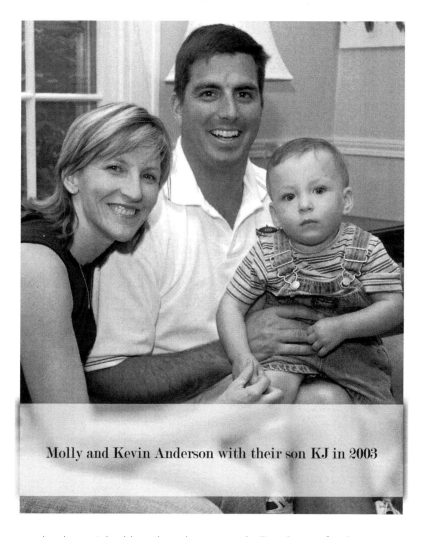

**Molly and Kevin Anderson with their son KJ in 2003**

that he weighed less than three pounds. First Steps of Indiana assessed KJ in the neonatal intensive care unit and connected the family with a LOGAN therapist, but he seemed healthy and went home without a diagnosis.

Eight months later, KJ was not developing normally, and he was eventually diagnosed with cerebral palsy. LOGAN was there to help.

"What impressed me most throughout all of KJ's early childhood intervention is that the LOGAN therapist came into his world," Molly said. "Jane Schmidt, the therapist, quickly understood the small circle of what KJ could get to and what he could do. She worked within that to increase his stamina and skills. Without the initial therapies early on, we would be looking at a totally different outcome for our son."

When it came time for KJ to attend school, the family chose to send him to St. Joseph Grade School in South Bend, a respected Catholic school in a multistory building constructed long before any thought to handicap accessibility.

They wanted KJ, who has two younger siblings, to experience the mainstream education—and they wanted the other children to experience him in their environment.

"KJ is blind to people's differences," said Molly, a member of the LOGAN Corporate Board of Directors who works as the Adidas representative for Notre Dame. "He has seen so many others with disabilities through therapies, medical visits, swimming, and other activities, yet he doesn't comment on others' disabilities.

"He has grown to have compassion. We felt that KJ attending this school was going to be better for KJ, for the family, and for the school. It was going to force them to reach out to and involve others because KJ was going to need their help."

She gave the school principal the book *Why Do I Walk With Canes, You Ask?* which the principal read to each class to increase understanding of KJ's situation. Two eighth graders were assigned to help him at the end of the day, a role that quickly became sought-after among the older students.

"As a parent, I see my role as trying to give my son the tools that he will need to handle what is ahead of him," Molly said. "I tell KJ that the attitude and the personality that you carry makes the difference. It is important to be a good person so that people will want to be around you for who you are.

"As a LOGAN parent, I think it's important for families to know that they don't have to go it alone, that LOGAN is there to help. I firmly believe in the saying that 'It takes a village to raise a child,' and that LOGAN plays a major part in building that village. LOGAN is very intertwined with our community."

## The Merluzzi Family

Bernadette and Tom Merluzzi had already decided to keep their daughter Msichana at home, rejecting a prominent doctor's recommendation for institutionalization after he diagnosed her seizures.

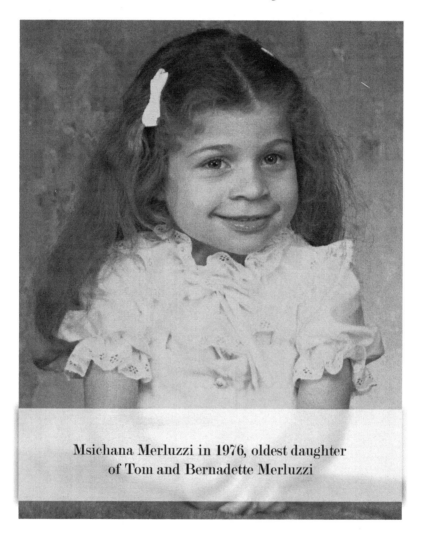

Msichana Merluzzi in 1976, oldest daughter of Tom and Bernadette Merluzzi

Connecting to LOGAN in South Bend, where they moved soon after Msichana was born in June 1974, meant that the choice would benefit not only their daughter but hundreds of other children in similar positions.

The support from LOGAN's HomeStart early childhood therapists who came to their home confirmed the Merluzzis' commitment, and their daughter went on to graduate from John Adams High School, crossing the stage to the cheers of her classmates in 1993.

Bernadette joined LOGAN's board in 1977, in time to win restoration of state funds for disability centers threatened by a budget crisis. With Executive Director Al Sonnoeker and state officials, she helped organize a public hearing at LOGAN Center that turned the tide.

Bernadette was also director of one of the first Parent Information Centers in the United States, started in South Bend, before she died in 1984.

Tom, a psychology professor at Notre Dame, was president of LOGAN's Protective Services Board when the Riverside Nursing Home crisis unfolded, and he held board meetings at nursing homes so members could see the low-quality care up close.

After a local hospital allowed a patient with mental disabilities to die for lack of measures to revive him— a "no code" policy— Merluzzi enlisted the help of Fr. James Burtchaell and Dr. Stanley Hauerwas of Notre Dame to train the board on end-of-life decisions.

"What I remember most is how respectful LOGAN was of the dignity of this man who had no family," Tom said. "LOGAN sought the best minds in ethics and theology to help train the Protective Services Board on end-of-life issues. Here was someone who had been forgotten. It was a testament to this man's life that LOGAN would never allow this to happen again."

chapter 6

# At Home

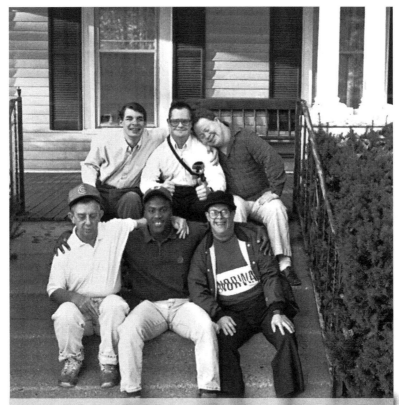

"We raised our children to value all different types of people, and we think it's a bonus that LOGAN moved into our neighborhood because it gave our kids a chance to meet someone and learn from them."

Peg Luecke

The first time LOGAN went to buy a house for a group home, leaders decided to hold a neighborhood meeting—not required for the purchase—to explain why they were coming to McKinley Terrace. The pastor who provided space in his church figured it would go fine. It didn't. While no one actually came out and said they didn't want people with disabilities living on their street, as longtime staff member Dan Ryan recalled, "this was an ugly meeting." Among the evasive objections, with parents of children who received LOGAN services present: the street was one of the last plowed in a snowstorm, making it difficult for emergency vehicles to get through. LOGAN withdrew its offer on the house.

Two months later, with an offer on a house in another neighborhood, the agency held another meeting attended mostly by families with young children. Someone speculated about the impact on property values, but a young mother rose to speak out and welcome the agency. LOGAN clients lived successfully in a house among those neighbors for 20 years. Looking back, Peg Luecke—a longtime LOGAN friend and wife of current South Bend Mayor Steve Luecke—is glad that she spoke out that evening. "We raised our children to value all different types of people, and we think it's a bonus that LOGAN moved into our neighborhood because it gave our kids a chance to meet someone and learn from them."

Group homes for people with disabilities were an important stage in the evolution of residential services for LOGAN clients, as for many such agencies across the country starting in the 1970s. The experience at Riverside cried out for new models to replace the institutional, often nursing home, warehousing of large numbers of people with disabilities in environments without sufficient services or expertise.

The LOGAN board started the experiment cautiously in 1974, renting instead of buying homes in case the model failed. The first purchase came in 1983, and, by the end of the 1980s, LOGAN owned and operated nine group homes in nine different neighborhoods. The board deliberately avoided clustering in a single neighborhood in order to increase the opportunity for citizens to live next door to LOGAN clients and get to know them.

Dan Ryan said LOGAN's integrative approach seems to be changing the climate in public places. He once took some group home friends out for a beer, and one especially loquacious resident with an unusual speech pattern insisted on sitting next to a businessman at the bar. Dan thought he should offer some explanation, but when he approached, the man offered to buy a round of beer. "My son lives in a group home in Illinois," he said, "and they never take them out and do cool things like this."

LOGAN built three new ranch-style group homes in the early 2000s, selling three of the older two-story group homes. The homes were designed

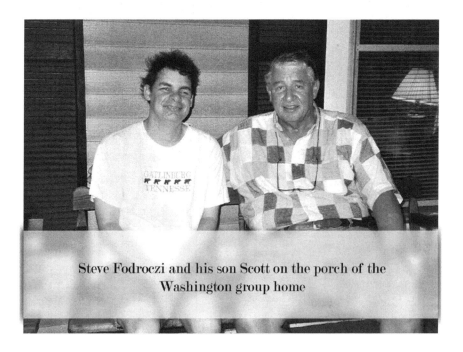

Steve Fodroczi and his son Scott on the porch of the
Washington group home

to meet the needs of aging residents with increasingly limited mobility as well as individuals with physical challenges who might come later. The agency expects to replace all of its group homes with the single-story style.

But the evolution was progressing to more ordinary residential settings for people with disabilities, including apartments with just two or three roommates. In 1986, the Supported Living Program started to support individuals living in apartment and private homes. This program transitioned in the early 1990s when LOGAN opened its first individual Medicaid waiver home, using state money to set up supported living options. Today, 70 clients live in such arrangements all over town.

The difference for the clients is striking. Steve Fodroczi, board president during the initial group home purchase, said that his son Scott still considered his parents' house "home" during the 10 years he lived with six other people in the house on Washington Street. As soon as he moved to an apartment with two friends, that became "home" and his parents' home became "folks' place." When Scott, who worked at Indiana University South Bend, became terminally ill, his roommates and caregivers told Fodroczi: "Scott's our family. He will stay with us as family as long as he can be with us." Scott died at the home surrounded by his LOGAN family.

Residential options provide a crucial answer for parents' fundamental fear: What will happen to my child when I die? In the old world of only at-home or institutional care, the solution seemed to be either an ongoing burden for the siblings or, sooner or later, the woefully inadequate and sometimes brutal life in a nursing home setting. With group homes and apartments, parents can already see the child living and thriving without them.

Sally Hamburg was already thinking of such a future for her son when she joined LOGAN's Residential Services Committee in the 1970s, when Joel was a toddler and the idea of group homes was in its infancy.

"It was really important to me that we look to the future," she said. "Parents don't live forever. What's going to happen to Joel when we're not here? We have to see that he has a life that is not totally dependent on us."

The road toward independence started while Joel was living at home and working at LOGAN Industries. Sally was taking him back and forth to work, but a staff person suggested that he learn to ride the bus. "I said, 'You have got to be kidding,'" Sally recalled, adding that she thought Joel lacked sufficient communication skills to manage transfers and other issues that might come up. "While his receptive language is fine," she says, "his expressive language skills are to the low end of the bell curve."

A LOGAN staff member agreed to ride with him, teach him the system, and evaluate when he would be able to manage it on his own. It took only three days. Joel was on a roll. He learned another bus route to his volunteer work at a hospital and yet another when he moved to a new home.

When he was in his 30s, Joel moved into an apartment with Jim, who grew up at NISH before he connected with LOGAN services and Dan Ryan, who became his guardian. Sally and Dan joked about becoming in-laws, and the group went apartment-hunting together. Jim, methodical and deliberate by nature, announced in the smaller bedroom of the chosen apartment: "This will be my room." Joel, exuberant and impulsive, was thrilled with his new home.

The day of the move, the group went out for pizza to celebrate, and the reality of the transition hit home for Sally: "I thought, 'This is strange. I'm going home and Joel is not coming with me.'"

Several days later, on the weekend, Sally was chatting with people in the apartment when Joel decided the visit should end—he had laundry to do. "He got up, opened the door, and said, 'Bye, Mom,'" Sally recalled. "That was the best feeling I could have had. He's very happy. It used to be I was attached to him at the hip. Now if I interfere with his schedule, he doesn't want any part of it." Jim took to calling Sally "Mom," and the Hamburg family included him on a trip to visit their daughter Ruthie in Las Vegas.

"They balance each other," Sally said. "Joel gets Jim going, and Jim gets Joel calmed down." When a third roommate moved in, she looked past her misgivings about the change because Joel and Jim didn't mind.

"The quality of Joel's life, which is my main concern, is wonderful," she said. "I am so glad we did what we did when we did it—letting go of Joel, trusting in LOGAN."

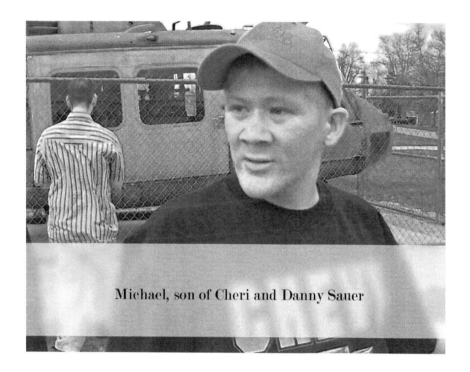

**Michael, son of Cheri and Danny Sauer**

## The Sauer Family

Michael Sauer started therapy with LOGAN when he was 11 months old, just six months after Cheri and Danny Sauer adopted him without realizing the severity of his developmental problems.

Although he'd suffered several ear infections, pneumonia, and, at nine months, a grand mal seizure, "it didn't change our mind," Cheri said. "We were in love with our son."

A social worker urged the couple to take Michael, who had earlier been evaluated in his foster home by a LOGAN HomeStart therapist, to LOGAN Center, where he received numerous therapies before entering the 2-year-old preschool class.

Michael was a member of the last graduating class from LOGAN's 3- to 5-year-olds before public education for such children from age 3 became a recognized right and schools started providing the service.

Michael was diagnosed with autism at age 9, when he first qualified for the Medicaid waiver, and underwent surgery for his digestive problems at 16. When he turned 18, he went into adult services at the Marshall Starke Developmental Center in Plymouth part-time while also receiving individualized habilitation through LOGAN.

When it came time for Michael to move, his parents made the difficult choice for him to join a LOGAN group home. The moving day, September 12, 2008, became an important date on the family calendar.

"Michael has made the transition really well," Cheri said. "When he visits our home now, he loves to check things to make sure that they are in their proper place. But it's apparent that he's ready to go back to his own home when the time comes. In his own words, it's 'Bye, Bye, guys!' when it's time to go back.

"I want to see him happy, and I see that now. We thought it would be very, very hard for him to make all these changes. But we're calm now and so is he. He's with the guys, and he loves that."

Meanwhile, Cheri, who started working in LOGAN's preschool while Michael attended, left for a while to concentrate on his care as his problems demanded. She returned to the preschool in 1990 and, when it closed, switched to Human Resources as an administrative assistant.

Now she provides administrative assistance to Building Blocks, the successor of Michael's first LOGAN program which gave him the start he needed in life.

chapter 7

# International
# Spotlight

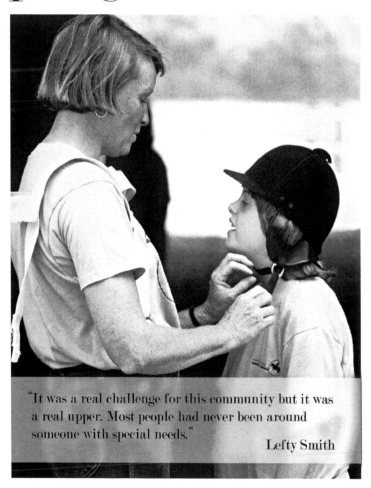

"It was a real challenge for this community but it was
a real upper. Most people had never been around
someone with special needs."

Lefty Smith

**N**egotiations with the Kennedy Foundation were down to the wire. South Bend had bid for the 1987 International Special Olympics Games, an event that had traveled all over the country every four years since its debut at Chicago's Soldier Field in 1968. Led by LOGAN and supported by the Chamber of Commerce of St. Joseph County and the University of Notre Dame whose facilities would become Olympic Village, the steering committee generated a written contract. The Kennedy Foundation had never signed such a thing and there was mounting suspense on both sides. Sargent Shriver called Fr. Ted Hesburgh, Notre Dame's president. Hesburgh asked Gene Corrigan, Notre Dame's athletic director, to call Dan Harshman, LOGAN's CEO, and Erv Derda, Games committee chair, to finish the negotiations. South Bend got a contract that protected the Council for the Retarded and the community from incurring debt as a result of the Games.

For the first time, the Games turned a profit, instead of the $1 million deficit that some earlier host cities had to cover. After paying expenses, the committee had enough to offer money to the next host city and launch the LOGAN Foundation.

The triple alliance—LOGAN, Notre Dame, and the Chamber of Commerce—was critical to the success of this international event. Notre Dame had a longstanding relationship with Special Olympics, reaching back to the days when Eunice Kennedy Shriver was organizing games for her sister Rosemary Kennedy.

Notre Dame football star Jim Mello, who had moved to Connecticut after his pro career, had gained fame for introducing athletics to a school for students with special needs, recalled Lefty Smith, a Notre Dame athletic official and longtime hockey coach.

"The Kennedys got in touch with Jim," Smith said. "Jim in turn went into the Washington area where they lived. Eunice ended up getting some kids in the neighborhood, and they started to set up an organized program for these mentally challenged young people."

That was the start of Special Olympics, which quickly spread to some 20 states. Another Notre Dame football star, Ziggy Czarobski, helped organize the first International Special Olympics in 1968 in Chicago, his hometown. Czarobski convinced the Conrad Hilton Hotel to donate rooms for the event and won use of Soldier Field from Mayor Richard Daly.

"There were a lot of Notre Dame connections to it," Smith said.

In 1982, Smith was president of the American Hockey Coaches Association when Canadian hockey player Larry McDonald was lobbying for the Special Olympics to add hockey. At the request of NBC President Dick Ebersol and his wife Susan St. James, Smith conducted a hockey clinic in Park City, Utah, and was invited to the 1983 International Special Olympics in Baton Rouge.

"I got down there and they put us with the celebrities," he said. "We had a chance to get deeply involved with a number of things in the games down there. We also got involved with the officers of the Special Olympics as well as the Kennedy family. When we were down at Baton Rouge, we knew they were looking for a place for the '87 games."

Together, Smith and Bill Locke, director of Recreation at LOGAN and area Special Olympics coordinator, decided to ask the Notre Dame administration to support a bid that would involve the campus as Olympic Village. Corrigan, Father Hesburgh, and Rev. Edmund P. Joyce offered their support.

After the Kennedy Foundation accepted the bid, there was a local effort to organize several Civitan clubs in Michiana, as the national organization was a strong supporter of Special Olympics. Civitan ended up donating

$1 million for the 1987 event. Locally, there was a strong effort to approach leading businesses and philanthropists to raise the remaining funds to reach the $5 million goal.

"Nobody here had ever heard of Civitan," Smith said, adding that Civitan International made significant financial contributions and their volunteers came from as far away as New Zealand. "We founded the clubs here. Some of them are still going. There were committees all over. People pitched in like it was going out of style. It took the whole town. Very few cities the size of South Bend would be involved in something like this."

Local families hosted celebrities and heads of state, welcoming Special Olympians from around the world. LOGAN volunteer Dick Gamble raised money to help a Tennessee Olympian's family of 17 children—including 15 adopted brothers and sisters, five with disabilities—attend the games to cheer on the oldest. The Expo Center at Saint Mary's College created an artificial snow mountain so that Olympians, including those from tropical climates, could experience snow and learn to ski. Three thousand athletes visited the St. Joseph County 4-H Fair.

Area garden clubs raised money for Bouquets for Victory presented to winning athletes. Twelve thousand bouquets were carefully arranged by a handful of women from boxes of red roses that filled the garage of Barbara and Steve Fodroczi, longtime LOGAN parents. St. Paul's Memorial United Methodist Church hosted a dinner for the Barbados delegation—22 athletes, seven coaches and sons, families and representatives. Church members waved Barbados flags at events and gave "Go Barbados Olympians" t-shirts to the athletes. The Italian delegation enjoyed a pizza party at Bruno's Restaurant. The Austrian delegation experienced a picnic with hamburgers, hot dogs, and apple pie.

The enthusiasm of the general community was matched by the university community.

"We couldn't have done it without Notre Dame being involved," said Dan Harshman. "We didn't have to go off-campus. It was a great Olympic

Village atmosphere. Notre Dame got us to the table." The university even delayed the opening of their fall semester for two weeks—an unprecedented action—so the games could take place.

The strong LOGAN-Notre Dame connection dated from the late 1960s, when LOGAN School was built across the street from the university campus. Students, many of whom did not have cars in those days, walked to volunteer at the center.

Decades later, that connection served to bring an international event that hosted 4,700 athletes from 70 countries and enlisted 18,000 volunteers, the vast majority from this community. The opening ceremonies, with 57,000 spectators and a total of 6,000 delegates, athletes, and coaches parading the field, were blessed by honorary chairman Fr. Ted Hesburgh before Whitney Houston performed. NBC carried the event on national television.

The Torch Run's final leg, from Soldier Field through 22 cities to South Bend, involved 57 police officers, part of a total 26,000-mile run by 30,000 officers from every state. Some 8,000 people lined the streets from Osceola through Mishawaka and South Bend to witness the torch on its way to the Notre Dame stadium.

"As we wrap up the final leg we begin history for northern Indiana," Notre Dame Basketball Coach Digger Phelps told the crowd. "We should be proud of what we've accomplished."

The success of the Special Olympics provided an economic, social, and public relations boon to the community. Hotels were filled for at least 30 miles. National television networks broadcast events and filled the airwaves with the heartwarming stories of athletes with disabilities from around the world. Eighteen thousand volunteers turned out for a multitude of jobs.

"We put together a company bigger than Studebaker in its prime," Erv Derda said. He met the president of Cessna in a Washington, D.C., hotel and arranged for 400 members of a Citation owners' club to provide free flights to South Bend for international participants once they reached U.S. soil.

Some 130 companies from 32 states donated their planes, pilots, and fuel worth $600,000 to bring athletes to the games, with arrivals from 16 cities at Michiana Regional Airport every three minutes in a six-hour stretch.

"It was a real challenge for this community, but it was a real upper," Smith said. "Most people had never been around someone with special needs." Thousands now had that experience.

The glow from the international event put LOGAN's mission in the forefront of this community, and the organization seized the opportunity to welcome volunteers and solicit support that would keep the momentum going. LOGAN launched the LOGAN Foundation as the agency's fundraising and development arm and hired its first volunteer coordinator to channel the heightened community interest and enthusiasm.

"The next time we open up a group home in a neighborhood or someone is interviewing someone with a disability for a job opening, I hope the impressions that were formed during the International Special Olympics will be remembered," Harshman told the local newspaper after the event. "I think many people are coming to the realization that people with disabilities can be good neighbors, that they can be good employees and that they can be strong assets for our community. That's what is really exciting. That's what really counts."

## Bill Locke

Bill Locke, LOGAN's recreation coordinator, felt the sting of discrimination that people with disabilities face routinely when he showed up at an underground Atlanta restaurant in the days when the Civil Rights movement was less complete.

The restaurant turned away LOGAN's Special Olympics basketball team, in Atlanta for a regional tournament, because Locke, his son Geary, and another player were African-American.

Just another reason for Locke, whose larger-than-life presence transformed LOGAN's recreation program and laid the foundation for the 1987 International Summer Special Olympics, to keep on fighting for equality on all fronts.

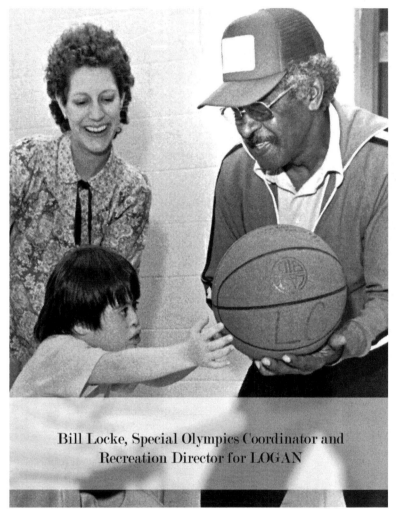

Bill Locke, Special Olympics Coordinator and
Recreation Director for LOGAN

"Bill was instrumental in growing the recreation program as well as personally helping hundreds of individuals with disabilities to grow," said Ann Lagomarcino, who worked with him on local and area Special Olympics programs before his sudden death, in his office, in 1984. "Bill's unconventional methods, creativity, and dedication made him a legend at LOGAN and in the community."

Locke, a college athlete hired as a social worker at LOGAN in the late 1960s, routinely wore his track suit and tennis shoes, ready for a pickup game of basketball, baseball, or golf at the drop of a hat. He quickly became recreation director.

His friends, who called him "Corky," became a base for Locke's far-reaching recruiting of donors, supporters, and volunteers for his recreation programs.

"Bill personally brought hundreds into the LOGAN mission as people came out of the woodwork for his events," Lagomarcino said. "Not a man for belaboring protocol, Bill was famous for his success in making things happen, lively and fun, with minimal resources."

Locke and his wife June had five children, including two sons with disabilities who became part of his entourage and a living example to other parents of the opportunities they should allow their children.

"Parents simply couldn't say no when Bill encouraged them to let go of their sons and daughters so they could experience new adventures," Lagomarcino said. "His sons were always very involved and Bill made sure that they worked just as hard and had just as many opportunities as any other child."

Opportunities abounded at the LOGAN Center on Eddy Street, where Locke opened the gym, cafeteria, and swimming pool for activities on evenings and weekends.

Locke's insistence on bringing the International Summer Special Olympics to South Bend, after he attended the event in Baton Rouge, launched the effort that culminated in the 1987 Games, three years after he died.

His son Geary lit the Olympic torch in his honor at the opening ceremonies in Notre Dame Stadium.

# chapter 8

# Raising Awareness

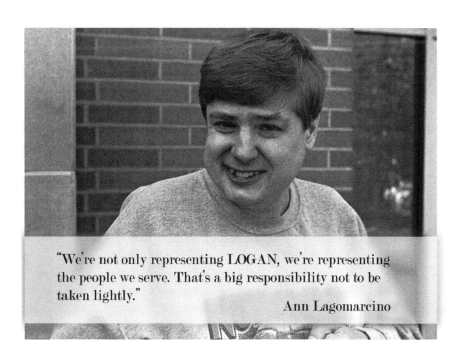

"We're not only representing LOGAN, we're representing the people we serve. That's a big responsibility not to be taken lightly."

Ann Lagomarcino

L OGAN launched its 60th anniversary celebration year on St. Patrick's Day 2010, with the annual Great LOGAN Nose-On Luncheon. Nearly 1,000 people filled a convention room at the South Bend Century Center for the event that has grown in 20 years to become one of the largest charity fundraising events on the city's calendar.

The Great LOGAN Nose-On, centered around a whimsical green foam ball formed to fit the face of school children, staff, clients, waitresses, bank tellers, and politicians, catches attention for the agency every year in the weeks leading up to St. Patrick's Day, in a community where Notre Dame makes any allusion to Irish appreciated. Green-dot yard signs sprout by the hundreds in neighborhoods and along thoroughfares, filling the landscape with LOGAN. A massive green dot adorns the LOGAN Center's portico-nose. Billboards of grinning clients in grayscale with the bright nose of green proclaim: You Nose It's Our Month! And everyone knows.

The luncheon, emceed by television anchor Maureen McFadden, who grew up playing with Irving Waxman, son of LOGAN founders, mainstreams the community's civic and business elite into the LOGAN world, where bank executives and elected officials share tables with clients and the volunteers who serve them. The crowd includes dozens of students sponsored to attend from more than 20 schools.

"We're counting on you to be the LOGAN advocates of the future," Dan Harshman told the students from the dais. "Be considerate of your fellow students at your school. Welcome them warmly to participate."

Support comes from the "A" list of northern Indiana institutions, including local and national businesses as well as individuals, with Irish-themed

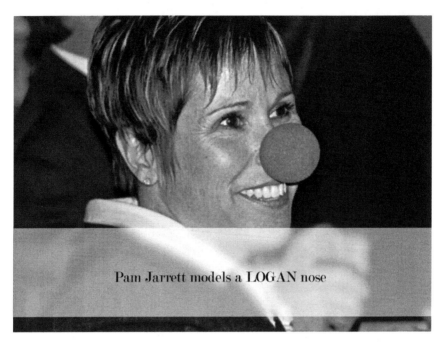

Pam Jarrett models a LOGAN nose

levels of participation from Pot o' Gold Presenting Sponsors and Shamrock Patrons to Blarney Patrons and Green Derby Table Sponsors.

For the 2010 Nose-On, South Bend chocolatier Mark Tarner created an edible version of the distinctive green sphere, a mint chocolate malt ball sold to benefit LOGAN and shared to sweeten the luncheon. Lou Pierce, owner of Big Idea Company, and his innovative team created "Yum," a playful video featuring the chocolate nose being enjoyed by clients, volunteers, families, staff, and the mayor of Mishawaka. LOGAN awarded its Noseworthy Award to the cast. Two dozen local businesses sold Nose-On merchandise, including the chocolate, and one company alone sold more than $12,000 worth of green accessories.

LOGAN honored longtime supporters Jan and Bob Hoenk and Karen and Mike Leep. Each received artwork by LOGAN client Martha McMillian. In addition to being the agency's largest family donors, the Leeps have provided employment for a LOGAN client at one of their car dealerships. First brought to LOGAN by their son Adam who has Down syndrome, the Hoenks have shown ongoing support as sponsors of LOGAN events and their support helped launch the first Team LOGAN for the 2006 LOGAN's Run.

FLAME, the only world-touring band composed entirely of people with disabilities, roused the crowd after lunch with a fast-paced set of seven favorites, from "Folsom Prison Blues" to "Sweet Home Alabama." The show of ability among the disability—two musicians use wheelchairs—gave sound evidence of the possibilities that places like LOGAN provide. Mike Seamon, assistant vice president of Events and Protocol at Notre Dame and chair of the LOGAN Foundation Board, reminded the crowd how it happens.

"There are people who need each of you, who need us, who need LOGAN," he said. "There is no greater calling in life than to help those who are in need."

Six decades after a handful of parents started putting on bake sales to pay a teacher for their children with disabilities, LOGAN has become one of the most respected and successful not-for-profit institutions in the region. That's because the drive for community awareness goes far beyond fundraising, vital as that is. The Great LOGAN Nose-On, LOGAN's Run, and other events that punctuate the year are an arm of the agency's advocacy mission, making sure that every person sees the smile on the face of disability and comes to understand the humanity and worth of every person living in their community.

Six decades after Joe Newman insisted that parents show pictures of all their children, even the photo in the back of the wallet, the whole city sees billboards of such children on its major streets. The breadth of activity reaches from filling a float with LOGAN clients that won Best in Parade at the city's St. Patrick's Day parade three years in a row to writing a column in the local paper detailing the social dangers of casually accepting comic use of "retard" in Hollywood movies such as *Tropic Thunder*.

The agency's public profile accelerated as a result of the 1987 International Summer Special Olympics Games. This Special Olympics event forever altered LOGAN's profile in the community and the public profile of people with disabilities. Thousands of neighbors saw, heard, cheered, and admired people with disabilities for the first time in their lives. Already-strong ties with Notre Dame deepened. Community volunteer leaders became board members. And LOGAN leaders learned to take their place among other prominent social agencies and charitable organizations in the community.

"This event brought us out," Harshman said. "After the games I think we really started to grow in terms of marketing and fundraising. We had never had anything close to professional marketing and fundraising. The first couple of generations worked at government revenue streams and grass roots fundraising."

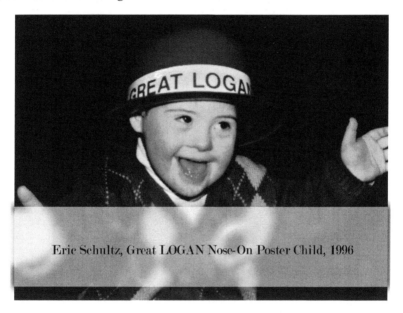

Eric Schultz, Great LOGAN Nose-On Poster Child, 1996

The early '90s was a turning point for LOGAN in the fundraising arena. The establishment of the LOGAN Foundation set the tone and the launching of the Great LOGAN Nose-On brought community energy and attention to the cause. The Nose-On took off during its first 14 years under Pam Jarrett, the agency's energetic development director from 1992-2006, who, with the Foundation Board of Directors, took fundraising to a new level for the agency. In 1999, with Tom Brokaw as the featured speaker at the Nose-On Luncheon, the event drew a record number.

When LOGAN entered a new level of fundraising, major community players taught the newcomer how to navigate the culture and collaborate with fellow leaders. The agency became more serious about marketing and telling its story effectively.

"The focus shifted to include major individual, corporate, and foundation gifts," Harshman recalled. "We had to build the right skills to compete. We needed to learn this piece about marketing. We had to build upon our reputation, which prompted us to reach out even more to tell our story. We were forced to develop professional skills in this area, an adjustment for all of us—board and staff. Yet our vigilance with respect to this process has had great value for us in connecting to the community, telling our story, and strengthening our organization. "

While the Great LOGAN Nose-On remains the signature event, others bring the mission forward throughout the year. Near the end of March, LOGAN hosts a Disability Awareness Fair for hundreds of fourth and fifth graders. Stations offer hands-on experience for them to better understand different disabilities and learn about technology and devices that help people overcome some of their challenges. The Fair thanks the students for their help with selling Nose-On merchandise and brings them face to face with the issues behind the noses.

In 2010, the Fair opened a new station that addressed the use of the R-word—"retard"—and asked the grade school students to sign a pledge never to use it in a hurtful way. Notre Dame students developed this station just weeks after participating in the national campus-based "Spread the Word to End the Word" campaign. At Notre Dame during that one-day campaign, more than 2,000 students signed the pledge, and hundreds wore student-designed t-shirts to promote the theme of respect.

LOGAN also hosts a Disability Awareness Event each year with Notre Dame and Saint Mary's College, featuring such speakers as Temple Grandin, an internationally renowned engineer who has autism, and performers such as Brittany Maier, an accomplished pianist who is blind and has autism. For the 60th anniversary, the event was a free FLAME concert, in addition to the band's Nose-On performance at South Bend's Century Center. More than 750 people attended, including students from grade school through college, professionals with their children, and LOGAN clients, families, and staff.

Once the seed of awareness is planted, who knows if and when it will take root and grow. While LOGAN promotes understanding and acceptance, the true measuring stick of inclusion lies in the lives of those sometimes forced to live life on the sidelines. One such story of an individual gives testimony to the advocacy behind LOGAN's mission.

"Heart and Soul" was the *South Bend Tribune*'s lead headline atop a football story and full color photo. It was the day before the 2007 home opener for Notre Dame football. But this story was not about Fighting Irish football. It was the story of LaVille, a small rural high school on the outskirts of town whose football team gave Trevor Langford the chance of a lifetime. Despite disabilities and a speech delay, Trevor had no problem communicating excitement about being part of the Lancer team. His teammates and coaches counted on Trevor to bring that enthusiasm to two-a-day practices, early game-day breakfasts, and ultimately to the gridiron Friday nights. When the opportunity presented itself to put Trevor in the game one night, the climate changed on the field, hard core competitiveness transformed to cooperation. The excitement of those on and off the field was off the charts as no. 70 "scored" a touchdown.

Keeping his highlight video, photos, and game ball close by, Trevor will tell you, "That were the best day of my life." His mother Jill, assistant development director for LOGAN reflects, "This is a shining example of how important inclusion is—not only for individuals with disabilities but for those who have the opportunity to be around them. The memories of these years will stay with Trevor for a lifetime and I am confident that his teammates will remember as well."

Now as parents of a young adult with disabilities, Jill and Jim Langford look to LOGAN to help them navigate the next phase of their son's life. According to his parents, that means Trevor being actively involved and not living life on the sidelines. According to Trevor, that could mean being part of yet another football team—one that practices under the Golden Dome. After all, LOGAN founders demonstrated the importance of dreaming big.

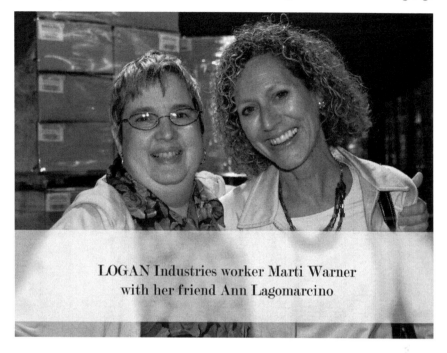

**LOGAN Industries worker Marti Warner with her friend Ann Lagomarcino**

## Ann Lagomarcino

Ann Lagomarcino was a teen when her mother signed her up to teach swimming to children with Down syndrome, providing the personal interaction that gave Ann a heart for people with disabilities.

"I fell in love with the kids and knew this was something I wanted to do," she recalled.

She earned a degree in recreational therapy at the University of Illinois at Champaign-Urbana and became activities director at a nursing home when she moved to South Bend in 1976.

Two years later, when a job opened at NISH, she went back to working with children with disabilities. The activities included swimming and gym play at LOGAN Center next door.

The first visit to NISH was overwhelming, Ann recalled: "I hadn't seen that many kids with that many significant disabilities in one spot before. When I got to know them as individuals, that faded away and I started loving them for who they were."

Eventually, she became volunteer coordinator at NISH, and earned a master's degree at the University of Notre Dame, focused on marketing classes. "I knew I wanted to work at LOGAN and I wanted to get more into community involvement," she said.

The opportunity came after the International Summer Special Olympics Games in 1987, where she had been an area coordinator with Bill Locke. LOGAN created a volunteer coordinator position to manage the surge in service that the event left in South Bend.

Now, as director of marketing, Ann manages the message—on billboards, at events, through news media and video—that communicates the breadth and depth of LOGAN's advocacy and service and cultivates its proud place in the community.

A decade ago, she coined the durable "Discover the Potential" brand, which turns out to include the potential of LOGAN and the potential of the community as well as the potential of the clients.

Fulfilling her role of increasing community awareness of both the mission and the people of LOGAN includes responsibility for three websites, support of several major fundraising events, coordination of volunteers, and oversight of relations with the media.

The work draws on the lesson she learned in the swimming pool years earlier—beyond the words, beyond the images, beyond the meetings and marketing, the fundraising and paperwork, the services and the lobbying, LOGAN is about real human beings.

"I always like to lead with the stories of people," she said. "Their stories speak for themselves—they are so compelling. I try to bring a face to the fundraisers. I like to invite people to come and get to know our folks. They are the best ambassadors for the LOGAN mission.

"I have a soft spot for the families. They encounter so many roadblocks, often getting overwhelmed, but they keep on trying. They amaze me. We want to offer them all that we can to help them overcome the tough spots. Their love for their sons and daughters keeps the passion of LOGAN alive.

"One of the biggest responsibilities I feel is that we're not only representing LOGAN, we're representing the people we serve. That's a responsibility not to be taken lightly."

chapter 9

# Part of
# the Team

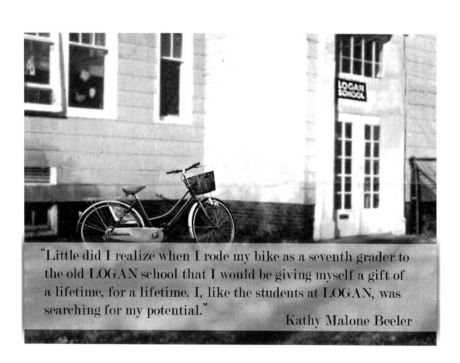

"Little did I realize when I rode my bike as a seventh grader to the old LOGAN school that I would be giving myself a gift of a lifetime, for a lifetime. I, like the students at LOGAN, was searching for my potential."

Kathy Malone Beeler

From the beginning, LOGAN families asked their friends to get involved in the movement to provide their children a decent life and an appropriate education. An eager cadre of community folks responded, helping renovate the first school building, raising money, spreading awareness that everyone should care about these long-neglected people in our midst, people who make us a better society.

As LOGAN grew, the army of volunteers grew as a vital support for the agency's expanding mission of service and advocacy. College students looking to get involved in the community and get off campus, younger students who befriended their classmates with disabilities, and adults moved by the needs of family friends have joined the cause. The growth in volunteers spiked when the 1987 International Summer Special Olympics Games brought LOGAN to the attention of thousands of Michiana people. Ongoing campaigns have built upon that awareness to continually attract new volunteers to the fold.

Through the years, volunteers have baked cakes and created candies, befriended children with disabilities and their siblings, taken adults on outings, planted gardens and painted schools, raised money for programs and buildings, and organized community-wide events like the Great LOGAN Nose-On and LOGAN's Run. Dedicated volunteers have offered their time and talents to oversee operations and fundraising from boards and committees.

Some volunteers served for years with no formal connections—such as Dick Gamble, recruited in the 1950s by a friend who worked at LOGAN Industries. For 40 years, Gamble, brought his business expertise to benefit fundraising, board, and committee activities.

Many community volunteers literally have grown up around LOGAN and remained active across the decades.

Kathy Malone Beeler started volunteering at the original LOGAN School when she was in the fifth grade, riding her bike over to help with the children because her classmate's brother Joey was in the school. "I remember becoming close with some of the kids and feeling that Joey and a couple of his buddies really looked forward to us returning on those Saturdays," she said. "Joey's ear-to-ear smile and outstretched arms directed to me as I parked my bike and approached the playground left an indelible mark on my heart and my mind." Beeler went on to volunteer at LOGAN Center on Eddy Street when she was a Saint Mary's College student and continued involvement as a volunteer and major donor in her adult years. She eventually chaired the LOGAN Foundation Board from 2004-2006, a time when the $6.7 campaign was underway to build the new LOGAN Center on Jefferson Boulevard.

Mary Jane Stanley followed the example of her mother Jane Kuzmitz, whose Service Guild was involved at the original school and went on to host monthly dances for decades at the LOGAN Center on Eddy Street. Mary Jane recalls going down the steep stairs to the basement classroom of the original clapboard schoolhouse on Logan Street, knowing that she would be greeted by her favorite student, Kevin Matthews. Years later, Mary Jane saw Kevin, a worker at LOGAN Industries, deliver the invocation at LOGAN's 50th anniversary dinner in the Monogram Room at Notre Dame. Always an avid LOGAN fan, Mary Jane continued her volunteer work, serving on committees, chairing the LOGAN Foundation Board (2000-2001), and helping to lead capital campaigns to raise money for renovations, expansion, and the new building.

While community volunteers were involved since the early days, the move to Eddy Street across from the University of Notre Dame in 1968,

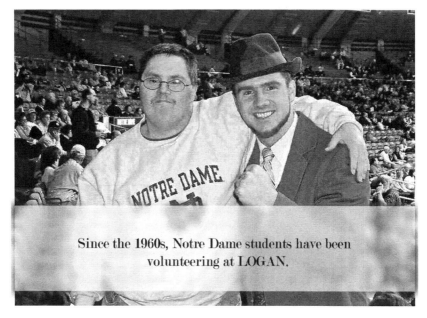

Since the 1960s, Notre Dame students have been
volunteering at LOGAN.

brought the LOGAN mission to the attention of socially conscious students who appreciated opportunities within easy walking distance.

"With Father Hesburgh playing Santa and Digger Phelps bringing his players and friends in for a basketball game with LOGAN clients at the annual holiday party, the partnership took off," Ann Lagomarcino says. "A core group started through the Linebacker Inn, an icon with its unique personality, for the Notre Dame and South Bend communities.

"Students became very involved in the Saturday Recreation Program, which actually started with Friday night bowling and dances and carried on into various activities on Saturday, including a fall football game, the Blue and Gold Game, and an overnight camping trip each spring. Word spread across campus—students brought their friends—and LOGAN became the place to meet people from the community and campus."

Dennis Stark, whose son Kenny was one of the first LOGAN School students, encouraged swimmers from Notre Dame, where he was coach, to volunteer in the LOGAN pool. The connection helped deepen the LOGAN-Notre Dame alliance. He was also involved in the local Special Olympics swimming program and on LOGAN boards and committees.

Some of the eventual staff, including Autism Center Director Dan Ryan, first linked to LOGAN as volunteers. Ken Hendricks, a LOGAN Protective Services Board member, and his wife Lori, a special education teacher whose brother had worked at LOGAN Industries, met at LOGAN when he was at Notre Dame.

"Ken simply wanted to get off campus, help out, and meet girls. His plan worked. " Lagomarcino says. "LOGAN was such a part of their lives together that the couple held a special wedding reception for their many LOGAN friends." Ken and Lori now have four children, including a child with special needs who has received services from LOGAN.

Soon after the International Special Olympics in 1987, LOGAN launched a Best Buddies program with Notre Dame and Saint Mary's College, a local chapter of International Best Buddies. This program started out with 15 LOGAN clients matched one-on-one with college students and swelled to more than 80 matches at one time.

"Friendships formed over the years and many students have kept in contact after graduation," Lagomarcino added. "Recently, Kate Mueller, one of the original LOGAN Best Buddies, proudly showed a photo of her Notre Dame buddy's third child. Kate attended her friend Julie's wedding and these women have stayed connected over the years even though they live in different states."

The LOGAN/Notre Dame Chapter of Best Buddies won the Chapter of the Year Award for Indiana in 2004 and International Chapter of the Year Award for the 2008-2009 academic year.

Best Buddies was such a success that LOGAN soon launched Super Sibs, a program to support the siblings of children with disabilities—and to address their parents' concerns about the challenges such family life presents. The "typical" children each relate to a college student who also has a sibling with special needs.

"The kids love to be around the college students and participate in all types of activities on campus," Lagomarcino said, adding that the popular program has a waiting list. "Interspersed throughout the year are Sib

Chats, which allow an avenue to talk about some of the issues of having a sibling with special needs with others who understand."

As mentors, the college sibs become role models for the younger sibs. Some sibling matches have lasted all four years of a student's academic career, a significant amount of time in the lives of the younger kids. The Go family started out with children in the inaugural Super Sibs group when their youngest, Veronica, who has Down syndrome, was just a baby. As Notre Dame students, some of the elder Go siblings went on to become college sibs in the LOGAN program. Now as a teenager, Veronica, a graduate of Building Blocks, is a regular participant in LOGAN's new recreation activities for school-age kids.

Other volunteer activities have developed across the years. "On a rainy, muddy October Saturday a couple of years ago, over 75 volunteers from the community, the Notre Dame St. Joseph Valley Alumni Club, and Congressman Joe Donnelly and his wife Jill gathered to build LOGAN's adaptive playground," Lagomarcino said. On the following Sunday, the Notre Dame Rugby Club spread mulch for hours to finish off the playground under the watchful eye of their coach, who made this project their mandatory conditioning for the day. To show thanks, LOGAN staff baked and packaged 20 dozen cookies for the next home rugby game.

Individual students work at LOGAN for both volunteer service and class credit. When Notre Dame's Center for Social Concerns created a service learning component that links community agencies with academic courses, LOGAN was one of the first organizations identified as a site where students could volunteer as part of their course work.

Notre Dame paid for a part-time position at LOGAN to work with professors and coordinate the student involvement through their coursework. LOGAN also became involved with preparing students and leading them on a spring break trip to the L'Arche communities of Toronto and Washington, D.C., where people with and without disabilities live together.

The connection with Saint Mary's College students has also been strong. Students from education and communication classes have been involved in programs through the Autism Center. Saint Mary's hosts an annual Halloween Trick or Treat event on campus for many LOGAN families and kids from Super Sibs.

Later, LOGAN raised its profile among Bethel College and Indiana University South Bend (IUSB) students. Bethel students recently formed Bethel Buddies, a popular group on campus that plans activities with teens and young adults who have Down syndrome. Students from IUSB turn to LOGAN for experiences that will provide credit for special education, psychology, and sociology classes. From universities and colleges across the Midwest, interns in counseling, social work, recreation therapy, special education, and occupational therapy come to LOGAN.

The mainstreaming of children with disabilities into elementary, middle, and high school classrooms has raised awareness among students in those schools who, in turn, volunteer in countless personal, informal ways as well as in organized programs. At the 2010 LOGAN Nose-On Luncheon, students from some 20 schools sat at sponsored tables and were recognized for their participation with LOGAN.

Volunteers come to LOGAN with all types of talents to offer. When LOGAN moved to its new home in 2005, the local Master Gardeners helped complete the elegant landscaping that surrounds the structure. Client Scott Fodroczi's mother Barbara introduced the gardeners to the agency. Chris and Bill Moyer, grandparents of a child with disabilities, meticulously maintain the flowers and shrubs that welcome visitors to the Center.

Ben Berger, a local golf pro who has a family member on the autism spectrum, used his athletic talent to raise money for the Autism Center. For five straight years, Ben made a major sacrifice for LOGAN, completing a one-person golf marathon from sunrise to sunset, 16 straight hours on the longest day of the year. Pledges for each hole, eagle, birdie, par, and bogey motivated Ben to play fast and play well. The first year, Ben surpassed his goal of 250 holes, completing 428 with impressive scores. In later years, Ben kept pressing for more, topping 600 holes at the grand finale in 2010 and earning wide attention from sports media while raising more than $150,000 for the *Sonya Ansari* Center for Autism at LOGAN over the five-year period.

LOGAN's broad opportunities for service attract a diverse set of volunteers committed to the cause. Some have become volunteer guardians through Protective Services, providing family for those who have none. Older volunteers help with mailings, gathering over coffee to stuff envelopes. Others open their homes and expansive lawns for a summer Garden Party that attracts over 300 guests and raises money for the Autism Center.

Whatever their talents, volunteers have always been welcomed into the LOGAN family, which finds its deepest roots in community people who care enough to give of their time, open their hearts, and share their energy to advance LOGAN's mission.

## Scotty

Francis Scott ("Scotty") was sure he wanted to work with a LOGAN client who could walk and talk, get involved in his family life, enjoy the outdoors.

Then he met Chris, who could neither walk nor talk, but whose bright smile and twinkling eyes won Scotty's heart. After three months of visits, Scotty became Chris' guardian through LOGAN Protective Services.

"I'm just a good friend of his," Scotty explained to a newspaper reporter some 20 years later, when he was 82 and Chris was 47.

Scotty, a World War II veteran who had been a salesman and food broker, filled his retirement years with about 40 hours of volunteer service a week, at the Center for the Homeless and St. Vincent DePaul as well as LOGAN.

He and his wife Maryvon had brought up four children, but he decided that he had room for more "family," a decision that led him to LOGAN Protective Services and to Chris.

"He understood the importance of becoming a voice for someone with a disability who had no one else to speak up for them,"

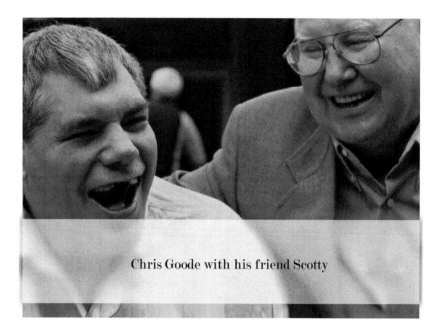

Chris Goode with his friend Scotty

said Ann Lagomarcino. "Gradually, Scotty came to understand even more—the importance of becoming family to someone who had no one involved in their life."

At first, he wanted to be a voice for someone with a voice, telling a LOGAN social worker that he hoped to bring the client home for dinner and conversation.

"The more time they spent together, the more Scotty felt the call to become Chris' guardian," Lagomarcino said. "It seemed that walking and talking wasn't all that important anymore."

Scotty was there for his friend through many transitions, such as when Chris moved from a nursing home to a group home. Scotty saw Chris gain new friends at LOGAN Adult Day Services and at Little Flower Catholic Church where they met every Sunday.

When Scotty died in 2006, Chris lost his best friend. But LOGAN Protective Services found another volunteer guardian for him, not to replace Scotty—no one could— but to make sure that Chris' voice is heard.

# chapter 10

# Those Who Serve

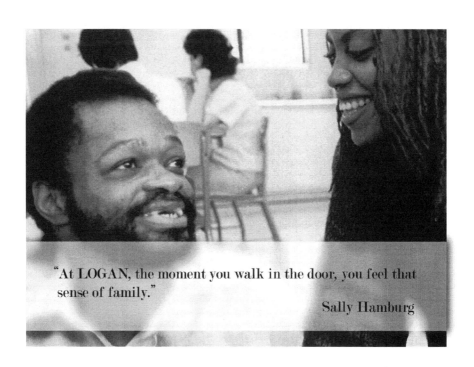

"At LOGAN, the moment you walk in the door, you feel that sense of family."

Sally Hamburg

Probably one of the best testaments to LOGAN staff is the way that they have weathered tough times as well as celebrated good times together over the years. Like other organizations across the country, LOGAN has endured belt-tightening periods and tough decisions. One such period in the agency's history was in 2003 when LOGAN faced fiscal challenges that precipitated the decision to sell the Eddy Street facility, its home since 1968, to Notre Dame. It was an emotional time. Ultimately, staff came together with parents and friends to dream of a new LOGAN Center that would far better suit the services now provided.

Following the role model of their founders, LOGAN faced this challenge by enlisting the help and support of others to build another new home for LOGAN. Once again, the community responded. Saint Joseph Regional Medical Center donated prime land and Ziolkowski Construction, architect and building contractor, donated the demolition of the 11-story building that stood on the lot. With these two gifts, LOGAN was well positioned to turn to the community and to foundations to raise the $6.2 million needed to build the new LOGAN Center.

As LOGAN prepared to leave its home of 37 years across from Notre Dame and occupy the new LOGAN Center in the summer of 2005, the staff for weeks took on the double duty of packing up for the one-weekend move while continuing to provide programs for clients. As the task progressed, the inevitable change became more and more visible—stacks of boxes in halls and corners—and a flood of emotions rose for the faithful old building, site of so many fond memories. As the final days approached, staff and clients took turns pressing their painted handprints on the hallway wall, marking their gratitude for the space where they shared so much life and love.

That was goodbye. All weekend, as they unpacked and prepared the new building, the staff steeled themselves for the Monday hello, wondering what the strange space would mean for their clients so attached to the routine and the familiar. Anxiety or excitement? Fear of the unknown or thrill at the new? Everyone on staff showed up that Monday morning to welcome the clients to their new home.

No worries. The clients knew, perhaps better than some of the staff, that LOGAN was not limited to the bricks and mortar on Eddy Street. They saw the faces of their friends, felt the usual welcome of the supportive staff that had earned their trust. They looked into the eyes of the people who had always looked at them as people of infinite dignity and worth, and they knew, whatever the changed address, they were home.

The friends of LOGAN staff say they must be special people, blessed with an extraordinary share of patience and compassion to interact day in and day out with people who have disabilities. But the people doing the work respectfully disagree. For them, the opportunity to represent the rest of us in meeting the needs of these people is a special vocation in its rewards, not so much its demands.

"They say, 'oh, that must be difficult,'" said Barbara Pickut, LOGAN Center's Adult Services manager. "It's intimidating if you don't know people. Once you get to know people, it's amazing to see how they express who they are and who they can be. I like to see how staff can accommodate to fit to one person's needs."

LOGAN's values—respect, kindness, honesty, loyalty, quality—took root in parents six decades ago and flourish today as the cornerstone of the organization, held up at staff orientations and posted to remind people at every turn in LOGAN facilities and group homes. The dedicated LOGAN staff knows that living those values requires seeing life through the eyes of individuals who must find alternate avenues to communicate and to navigate their world. It takes creativity and problem solving, patience and compassion.

**110**

Life in the world of people with disabilities comes with celebrations and sorrows, successes and setbacks—like the rest of life. Those who have chosen to work in that world seem to have accepted that reality ahead of time, a lesson everyone must eventually learn no matter where they work.

The vocation permeates LOGAN in complementary and overlapping ways. Some staff, such as Autism Center Director Dan Ryan and Children's Services Director Reecie Verslype are also volunteer guardians. Dan has helped Jim and Reecie has helped David, both men with Down syndrome, through changes across their lives. As guardians *and* friends, they celebrated with Jim and David when eventually the two, who grew up at NISH and lived in group homes, moved into their own apartments.

Others, such as Cheri Sauer, Building Blocks administrative assistant, and Annie Micinski, service soordinator, give back to the organization that has supported them in circumstances with their own children. Anne Kellenberg-True, director of Protective Services, adopted a young girl with Down syndrome born on an Indian reservation in California, adding a lively fourth child to her family.

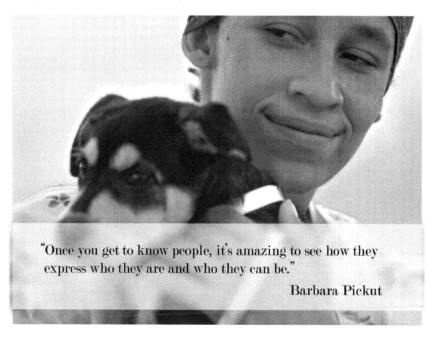

"Once you get to know people, it's amazing to see how they express who they are and who they can be."

Barbara Pickut

One couple met and fell in love at LOGAN. Tim Silverberg, a newly hired recreation assistant, met Cherry, a volunteer at the summer day camp, before she joined LOGAN as an employee. Truly a LOGAN love story, their courtship centered around recreation events and ultimately led to their wedding in 1975. Their two sons were raised around LOGAN and one now works there. Together, Tim and Cherry combine for a total of 60 years of employment with LOGAN.

Staff members find creative ways to befriend clients. Tim Silverberg, the agency's longest-term employee at 37 years' of service, takes his buddies golfing. Protective Services caseworker Sue Correa takes her friend Martha on trips and encourages her artistic talent. Sales Manager John Ayers, an icon at LOGAN Industries since the 1970s, finds ongoing ways to show his personal interest in each of the 160 workers in the workshop.

Sally Hamburg, whose son Joel is in LOGAN's Supported Living Program, believes the staff's dedication enhances the quality of life for Joel and his household.

"It is clear that Jeff Johnston, director of Supported Living, really knows and cares about the individuals served by the program and interacts with them on a level that is an extraordinary example of what LOGAN should expect of all staff," she said. "Jeff Reed as program coordinator for 'the guys' is phenomenal. It is clear that he knows Joel and his apartment mates quite well—their likes, their dislikes, their quirks, their needs, and what's in their best interests. He is so very dedicated to them as well as to the other staff that he supervises and from whom he expects quality treatment for 'the guys.' Not only is Jeff involved in the lives of Joel and his apartment mates, but so is his wife, who is often a volunteer participant in their activities and their celebrations."

The accounting staff also enjoys getting into the mix. Director of Finance Sharron Carter makes sure her employees are in tune to the mission. Among other things, the department hosts Bingo at the annual LOGAN Industries picnic. "It's amazing how we feel part of the LOGAN family," she said. "You don't have to be just on the program side. Accounting staff are now known as the Bingo people. The staff needs to see the faces of the people we serve so we remember that we all work here for a reason."

Sharron's work has brought her whole family into the LOGAN family. Her husband Mike, who had his own construction business, became director of Maintenance in 2005. Their daughters, Allyson and McKenna, are regular volunteers who pull their friends in to help. As Sharron sees it: "LOGAN gets in your blood. It's certainly gotten into the Carter blood now."

Sharing in the commitment and care for people with disabilities fosters a special closeness for staff. In 1997, Barb Deskovich, LOGAN's chief operating officer, died suddenly at the age of 38, surrounded by coworkers at the annual Thanksgiving staff luncheon. The overwhelming grief was felt throughout the organization as staff sought comfort from each other. Her office, left untouched for months, served as a reminder of a respected leader. Today, the LOGAN values, which she helped to create, serve as a memory to staff who knew her well.

A fountain in memory of Jerry Oberly graces the gardens at LOGAN Center. Jerry, a LOGAN employee for 30 years, passed away shortly after the move to the new LOGAN Center. He took a personal interest in the flowers surrounding the LOGAN buildings and group homes, often donating specialty items for the gardens.

This close sense of family extends beyond the circle of staff to include families and volunteers. Mary Ann, youngest child of Rocky and Rosetta Ferraro, was blind and had severe disabilities when she came as a child, and she benefited from LOGAN services into adulthood with the support of her loving parents. In 2005, Mary Ann and Rocky died within four months of each other, and a group of staff members and mothers close to the family organized a Lunch Bunch to support Rosetta—an ongoing event that Rosetta soon insisted on hosting with her Italian cuisine.

For Annie Micinski, now service coordinator for adults, the first contact with LOGAN came in 1980 when her daughter Jessica was diagnosed with cerebral palsy. The pediatrician, unsure whether her daughter would ever walk or talk, suggested she call LOGAN. The first response from

LOGAN was, "Let's get some help in there and see what we can do for your daughter," Annie recalled. "It was the first hope I'd had since she was diagnosed and probably the first time I'd smiled in a while."

Jessica received services at home until she was 3, then went to preschool at LOGAN until she was 5. Her younger sister Nichole came to preschool with her in the integrated classroom that always included at least two community children without disabilities. "LOGAN has always given people chances—not only people with disabilities, but also employees. The people I work with are absolutely amazing. I have learned so much from my coworkers. LOGAN has taken care of me and my family all these years."

LOGAN staff has multiplied since the day that the original LOGAN School opened with two teachers. With more and more parents bringing children with special needs, the staff and volunteer sides each grew exponentially. By its 60th year, LOGAN employed 362 people, including nine with more than 30 years of service and another 20 with more than 20 years.

In 2003, Herman Beutel established the Beutel Family Award in honor of his wife Rosemary, a leader of the Adult Day Services Parent Group for many years. Their daughter Susan had been involved with LOGAN from childhood until her death as an adult, and the family valued the staff's support. The award goes to an employee who exemplifies LOGAN's values. Herman and Rosemary have died, but their son Craig presents the award at the Employee Recognition Luncheon each year.

Throughout the years, parents have showed their appreciation for staff in many different ways, supporting the very people who have in turn supported their sons and daughters. Harshman reflects on one such parent who continually reminded the organization that their quality staff was a real treasure. Wart Donaldson, an active board member during the 1980s and '90s whose daughter Kay still receives services today, always seemed to be on the pulse of what was going on with the staff. In a very productive way, Wart would approach Harshman when he thought it best for LOGAN's leader to know what was on the minds of his employees.

"LOGAN is more than an agency that provides services for people with developmental disabilities—it is a family," Sally Hamburg said. "Therefore, it is important for the staff to feel that sense of LOGAN family, that they are just as vital as the clients, parents, volunteers, and donors. What drives the services and maintains the quality of those services are the people that provide them from the top down. The staff sees that it's not just a job; it is being a part of the lives of the clients. They believe in the individuals they support and understand that you never reach your full potential. Because if you do, you stop growing.

"Even staff who are not directly involved with clients are reminded daily of the LOGAN mission. Without those people and the leadership that supports them, LOGAN would not be the place that it is. When you don't have that, there's a disconnect between what happens and what you believe should happen. At LOGAN, the moment you walk in the door, you feel that sense of family."

## Dan Ryan

Two months before Dan Ryan was born, his mother's best friend gave birth to a son, Peter, with cerebral palsy. The boys were such close playmates and friends that Peter's mother would call Dan to help convince Peter that his hearing aids were cool enough to wear.

Certain that his career would involve working with people with disabilities, Dan earned a psychology degree from the University of Notre Dame while volunteering at NISH, next door to LOGAN Center.

When he graduated, Dan went to work at NISH and won a grant that allowed two teens from the Center to live with him in an apartment on Notre Dame Avenue while he was in graduate school. For two boys who had grown up in an institution, this was an incredible opportunity. It also was ideal for Dan who had gone back to graduate school.

Later, Dan was living in a L'Arche community in Toronto when LOGAN's CEO Dan Harshman hired him as residential director in 1978. In his dozen years in that role, LOGAN started buying group homes and setting up supported living situations in apartments.

After the 1987 International Summer Special Olympics Games, Dan became director of Special Projects at LOGAN and coordinated

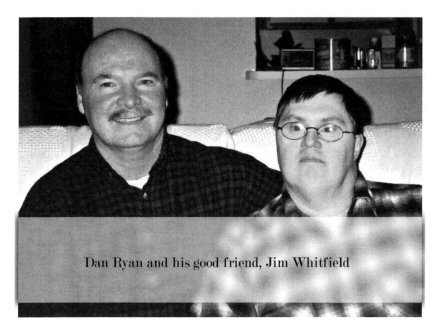

Dan Ryan and his good friend, Jim Whitfield

a national conference in South Bend tied to an initiative on employment for people with disabilities. He then became director of Education, then director of the Resource Center, and, in 2004, director for the Autism Center.

Meanwhile, Dan is the volunteer guardian for Jim, a friend from the NISH days who was with him in the Notre Dame Avenue apartment, through LOGAN Protective Services.

"The relationships with clients, co-workers, and families have kept me at LOGAN for more than 30 years," he said. "I find a sense of pride in the fact that LOGAN is admired in our community as a quality organization."

chapter **11**

# A Growing
# Challenge

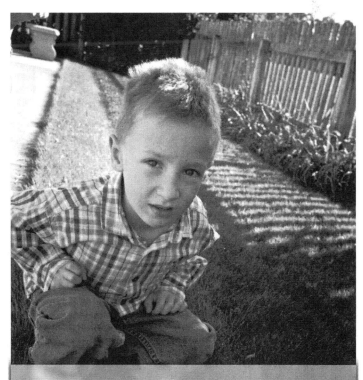

"At first... it's like losing a dream. As you get into it,
you discover your child is fabulous. And you want the
world to be better for him."

Kristen Hill Hake

A rapid increase in the number of people diagnosed with autism and Asperger's syndrome poses one of the biggest challenges LOGAN faces in its 60th year. The Centers for Disease Control estimates that 1 in 110 individuals will be diagnosed on the autism spectrum, compared with 1 in 1,000 just 20 years ago. As usual, LOGAN is leading in the effort to provide services to those families. A wing of the new LOGAN Center now houses the *Sonya Ansari* Center for Autism—concrete evidence of LOGAN's commitment to serve these people and their families.

The challenges stem not only from the dizzying explosion of need but also the sometimes difficult behaviors, unique learning styles, and communication problems that make it difficult for these individuals to fit into typical classrooms, jobs, and general life. Autism has gained national attention which has shed light upon the disability that is often more subtle and less recognizable than other disabilities such as Down syndrome and cerebral palsy. Driven by the need, LOGAN stepped up to offer resources and eventually services to families, despite limited available funding.

As advocates, LOGAN decided to supplement the information, resources, and support that public agencies such as school systems could offer. Dr. Tom Whitman, a Notre Dame professor who had written a book about autism, proposed a regional autism center to address the accelerating needs. Whitman involved his psychology students directly with children on the autism spectrum, using Applied Behavior Analysis techniques with encouraging results for local families. LOGAN gathered allies, including Notre Dame, Saint Mary's College, Memorial Hospital, Saint Joseph Regional Medical Center, South Bend Community School Corporation, and Joint Services for Special Education for School City of Mishawaka/Penn-Harris-Madison School Corporation to launch the Regional Autism Center in 2004. Dan Ryan was named director, and the center was a one-room resource library in the LOGAN Center on Eddy Street. Memorial Hospital paid the director's salary for the initial years.

Six years later, LOGAN shoulders full responsibility for the Autism Center, which has expanded not only into a full range of services but also into training for families, professionals, schools, and community organizations such as the Center for the Homeless and police departments. The *Sonya Ansari* Center for Autism, rather than adopting one treatment modality, tailors its approach to fit different individuals with autism spectrum disorders based on how the disorder manifests itself and the person's family situation.

That means the Center's services include a range from behavioral therapy and consultation to social skills classes, recreation activities, and summer camps. The Center offers the PLAY Project (Play & Language for Autistic Youngsters), a highly effective approach that requires specialized training of therapists. Renowned expert Dr. Richard Solomon created the PLAY Project as a practical implementation of Dr. Stanley Greenspan's Floortime Model, a highly successful approach that teaches parents and caregivers how to play with the child in order to gain therapeutic results.

In addition, the Center's certified behavior consultants use a combination of Applied Behavioral Analysis and parent training to work with individuals with autism who struggle with "triggers" in their environment that interfere with their ability to function in daily life. These therapists work in homes, schools, or wherever needed to teach appropriate behaviors. They also problem-solve, dealing with the stimulation, noises, food sensitivities, change in routine, anxieties, or obsessions that interfere with the person's ability to function.

The first clients of the Autism Center were children, but services soon expanded to teens and adults, with counseling services, a teen club, and a young adult group interested in advanced education and skills for jobs and independent living. Dan Ryan has been appointed to the Indiana Interagency Autism Coordinating Committee (IIACC), a state-wide committee charged with designing a comprehensive system of services for individuals on the autism spectrum and making recommendations to the Indiana Autism Commission for its lobbying efforts.

Responding to the interest in higher education, the Center developed an online resource tool featuring midwest colleges and universities that provide additional support for students with learning challenges, not just for those on the autism spectrum. This led to LOGAN's first College Fair, with 20 colleges and universities present.

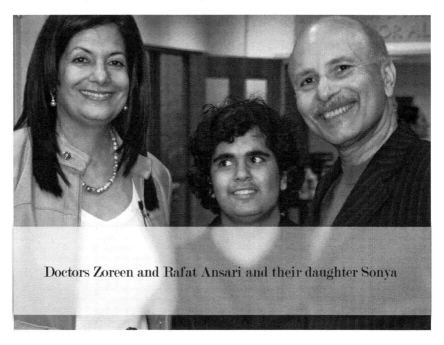

Doctors Zoreen and Rafat Ansari and their daughter Sonya

The philanthropy of Drs. Zoreen and Rafat Ansari in honor of their daughter Sonya—whose name the Center took in 2008—has supported rapid growth for advocacy and services. The Center has a team of dedicated employees and serves more than 250 people in eight counties, reaching into Michigan for the first time in LOGAN's story. The burst of activity in the new field comes as an expression of LOGAN's founding commitment to serve people with all developmental disabilities.

"We had to evolve and change," Harshman said. "We made the decision to re-identify ourselves as serving a broader spectrum. With autism identified as the single fastest-growing disability, it was important to grow in new ways to reach out to this demographic."

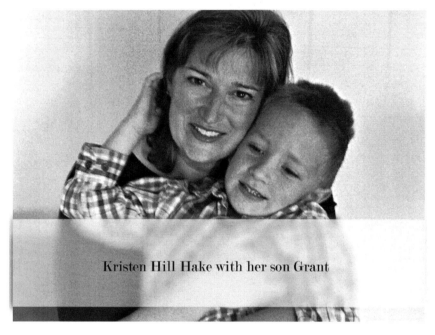

Kristen Hill Hake with her son Grant

## Kris and Grant Hake

When Grant Hake was diagnosed with autism at 18 months, some 10 years ago, his mother Kris started thinking decades down the road.

"When you have a child with a significant disability, the thing that keeps you up at night is 'What's going to happen when I'm gone?'" she said. "It became very important for me to become involved in LOGAN because this is my son's future."

After the shock of the diagnosis, Kris quickly learned the upside of raising a child with autism.

"It's devastating," she recalled. "You want your child to achieve everything they can in life. It's like losing a dream. As you get into it, you discover your child is fabulous. They don't have an agenda. They're not manipulative. You want the world to be better for them.

"Everyone that knows someone with a disability realizes what a blessing they are and how valuable they are in our world. They are an absolute joy. My son is just the light of my life. I want to make sure our society is a better place for him."

Society is better because of Grant, who tutors his elementary-school classmates and helps them experience diversity.

"Not only is my child helping them with their math, but it's teaching them that everybody is different," Kris said. "The sooner you learn that, the better off you are. Autistic kids can be very bright. But socially, there can be lots of challenges.

"I love the whole philosophy of inclusion. It's beneficial to everybody. We're almost seeing a civil rights movement for disabled people," she said, adding that the interactions enrich society: "Don't change me. Just accept me. Different is OK."

LOGAN's focus on ability, not just disability, and its settled presence in the community give confidence to parents who understand their critical role in the agency.

"The parents are given a voice as to how we want to see the future," she said. "I don't know how far Grant's going to go. If he needs to have supported living, I would like for LOGAN to be involved in that. I see him maybe working at LOGAN Industries in some capacity. He could be a number cruncher."

Whatever Grant's future, Kris knows LOGAN will be there for him.

"We're not going to be here forever, but LOGAN will hopefully continue on and on and on," she said. "It means so much to families to know there's going to be a game plan for our children. We know LOGAN is established. They're not going away.

"We're carrying on the mission of those original parents. They were our mentors. They're passing the torch to the newer generation of parents who have that continuity."

chapter **12**

# A Life
# Well Lived

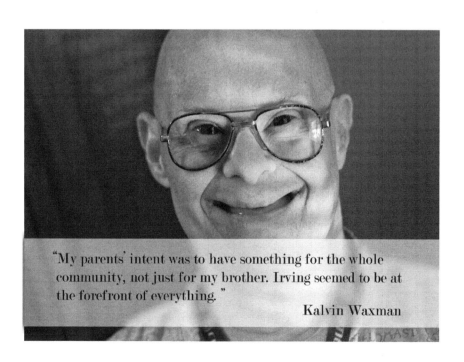

"My parents' intent was to have something for the whole community, not just for my brother. Irving seemed to be at the forefront of everything."

Kalvin Waxman

People with disabilities have taught LOGAN the fundamental value of every individual life and the fundamental interdependence of the entire human community. As Joe Newman always preached, no bright line separates people with disabilities from the rest of society, and our dependence on others varies only in degree. Within LOGAN, a Human Rights Committee oversees how the staff respects and cares for clients. Within society, LOGAN gives them voice.

"No one is able to completely take care of themselves," Dan Harshman said. "We need to step up to help those with disabilities who, like most of us, cannot go it alone. It's not just a matter of whether they have an education, a job, an apartment. It's also a matter of whether the fabric of their life is whole and complete. Are the right people around them? We're all going to need something, whether it's from birth or because of an accident or old age. At some point we'll all be calling on society."

Across its whole 60-year existence, LOGAN has provided such a life for Irving Waxman, son of founders Marion and Sol Waxman, a leading inspiration for the founding of LOGAN in the first place.

Doctors in 1946 advised the Waxmans to institutionalize their son, Irving, who had Down syndrome because he probably wouldn't live five years anyway and would disrupt the lives of their two other children.

Instead, the Waxmans, who had just moved to South Bend from Chicago to leave the painful memories of Irving's namesake, Marion's brother who died in World War II, helped launch LOGAN to make sure their baby would have the richest life possible.

The family, with relatives in South Bend, moved into an apartment above their W&W Food Market near downtown South Bend. The grocery consumed Sol's week. Marion learned to drive. The mission to create opportunities for Irving and others like him consumed Marion's week.

Marion and Sol took Kal, five years older than Irving, and their daughter Diane to look after him in the old building at LOGAN Street and Lincolnway where they were forming a school.

"I remember when this group of parents that my mom and dad were part of first rented space at what became known as LOGAN School," Kal recalls. "The building was not evidently being used, and they arranged to rent the building at that time, starting in the basement.

"Mom and Dad were either involved with meetings or helping clean up so they could get going in that facility. We went along for the ride. Babysitters weren't as common at that time. That was my contribution, I guess, to play with Irving at meetings while they were doing important things.

"It was a constant, never-ending process. Mom and Dad were very attentive to my needs and Diane's needs, but Irving had needs too. I don't think we ever felt left out or unattended. We were participants."

Ada Marker was the first teacher at the school, hired on faith when the group had a few dollars on hand and some fundraising schemes in mind. Kal remembers stuffing envelopes for the annual solicitation, and he remembers the cakewalks at the Fun Fair in the school that raised both money and community awareness.

Mostly, he remembers his parents' drive to provide for Irving.

"They were told he would probably not live beyond the age of 5," Kal says. "They were told to institutionalize him. There was no way they were going to do that.

"We have gone through the whole process from beginning to end. It wasn't their intent just to have something for him. It was for the community, too. Irving seemed to be on the forefront of a lot of things."

Irving was working for LOGAN Industries even before the workshop was moved to High Street, then rode the bus to the new manufacturing facility, built in 1981 in an industrial park north of town.

128

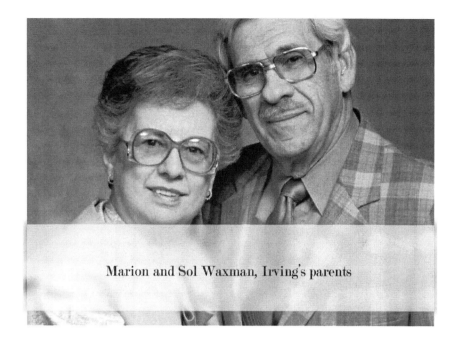

Marion and Sol Waxman, Irving's parents

He moved from his parents' home in the early 1980s, when he was nearly 40, to the group home on Washington Street where some LOGAN clients lived, a well-recognized group waiting at the corner of Jefferson and Eddy streets for the bus to LOGAN Industries.

"That was a big step for Mom to let him go from her house," Kal explains. "Every new step was a big thing, like the first time he rode the bus by himself to go to the workshop. She went with him at first. Sometimes he didn't get home on the bus. Where do you start to look? He could have gotten off anywhere. He was always very social and aware of people and comfortable being around people."

Sometimes Irving would deliberately get on a different bus for the change of scenery. Sometimes he would ride to the end of the line and come back. Sometimes he came home in a police car, yet another adventure.

"When it came time for him to move out, they had experienced little steps along the way to make that big step a little easier," Kal says. "It was still huge."

Irving's nickname "Butch" was made famous because of his friendship with Digger Phelps, who coordinated a basketball game every December between LOGAN and Notre Dame players. "Butch" was an icon for the tradition because somehow every year he was the player who managed to pull out the LOGAN win.

Meanwhile, Irving became an avid Special Olympics participant, taking third place in swimming at the inaugural International Special Olympics—tracking Kal, somewhat belatedly, in an athletic career.

"If I was able to do these things, he thought he should be able to do them, too," explained Kal, who coached high school wrestling for 20 years. Sol brought Irving, who had grown up watching TV wrestling with his grandmother, to the matches.

When LOGAN was closing the Washington Street group home, a friend of Kal's from Camp Eberhart rented his house in town to Irving and the families of two other men who needed a place. The families had known each other for years and worked together, and with LOGAN, to provide appropriate supports for the new home. After several years, negotiating the stairs to the second floor became a problem and the trio moved to an apartment.

Advocacy was a significant part of Marion's involvement with LOGAN. She became a vocal advocate for families to transition their children with disabilities into LOGAN residences as soon as practical, before the death of a parent forced the move amid additional traumatic circumstances. The longtime LOGAN board member and former chair labored over her speeches to state legislators on behalf of people with disabilities. Her job as bookkeeper for Ziolkowski Construction inspired the company's generous work for LOGAN in the construction of its new building. "You just couldn't say no to Marion," explained owner Ben Ziolkowski.

She also insisted, quietly, that Irving get the chance to participate fully in all of life, including the synagogue rituals so meaningful to him.

"She was so matter-of-fact about who Irving was," Kal says. "Marion wasn't one to stand on a soap box and say, 'I've got this kid with a problem.' We went to services as a family. Irving was accepted as part of the family of the synagogue," opening the Ark to present the Torah scrolls. "He took that honor very seriously."

"You have to know how tenacious Marion was to see to it that Irving would have positive experiences—maybe not be able to do everything every other kid would be able to do, but try his wings anywhere he chose," explains Kal's wife Bonnie.

The doctors were wrong about Irving's life—its quality as well as its longevity. Even Marion, determined as she was, marveled at the breadth of accomplishments, far beyond what she could have expected in 1946. A plaque at LOGAN reads:

"Marion and Sol Waxman had a vision for their youngest child, Irving, who was born with Down syndrome. They saw a bright future for their son, which, back in the 1950s, was not always a possibility for children with mental retardation. Marion and Sol wanted Irving to have opportunities like their other children had. They would not accept doors being closed to him simply because of his disability.

"The Waxmans were true pioneers and champions, on behalf of their son and all children with developmental disabilities. They encouraged other parents to work together to achieve what they all hoped for—the chance for their children to be participants, not just spectators, in life. Hence, LOGAN was born.

"Marion and Sol often said they never imagined that Irving or LOGAN could accomplish so much. They took pride in Irving's accomplishments, as well as in LOGAN's. Yet, they always encouraged LOGAN to do more to discover the potential in every person."

The doctors also were wrong about Irving's impact on his siblings.

"We were part of the support team," Kal says. "Our kids are the same way. Irving's part of the family. He's part of who we are, and who we became."

As Irving grew up, so did LOGAN. By the time LOGAN was celebrating its 60th anniversary, Irving had enjoyed its education, day programs,

Special Olympics, camping weekends with Notre Dame students, 40 years of work at LOGAN Industries, three different residential arrangements, and unwavering support from the ever-expanding circle of LOGAN clients, friends, volunteers, and staff.

LOGAN workers helped his siblings, who became his guardians, transition Irving to nursing home care, because of advancing Alzheimer's disease. On August 22, 2010, Irving died at the age of 63.

His full life, both a cause and a consequence of the LOGAN experience that has enriched thousands of other lives, stands as a symbol of the agency's mission, where advocacy and service combine in the interest of the human person.

chapter **13**

# Future
# Challenges

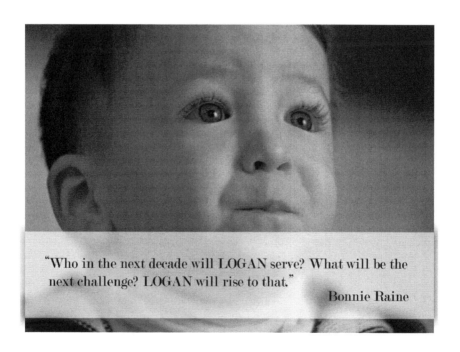

"Who in the next decade will LOGAN serve? What will be the next challenge? LOGAN will rise to that."

Bonnie Raine

On October 23, 2005, Joe Newman delivered the dedicatory address for the new LOGAN Center on Jefferson Boulevard in South Bend, telling the hundreds gathered to stay faithful to the founding vision. "With every move of the mission to other buildings went the name LOGAN, just as it has come to this new home," he said. "For now, the name of LOGAN and its mission has acquired meaning. Yes, the name has become a legacy and its mission a commitment."

Recounting the LOGAN story, Newman said: "Many years ago in several houses in this area, there were children who had needs that were being ignored. The doors of opportunity for these children were locked. The parents in those houses had hopes that these needs could be met and those locked doors opened. Those mothers and fathers met and hoped and planned together. And with determination, those hopes became a vision. They were so proud and so anxious to make known their vision that they painted the old schoolhouse on Logan Street a brilliant white. And to demonstrate their determination, they placed a big sign that almost shouted: 'LOGAN School for Retarded Children.' That is what their children were called back then."

When it came time to build a new home, the name LOGAN—like the purpose—remained, long after the move from the original schoolhouse in Mishawaka where Family and Children's Center now stands. Grassroots efforts of family and friends combined with government grants and community donations to raise money for a state-of-the-art school building built in 1968 across the street from the University of Notre Dame, in the block with the Northern Indiana State Hospital for children with developmental disabilities.

Like the larger Civil Rights movement that it has tracked for 60 years, the movement for the disabled in general—and LOGAN in particular—has enjoyed astonishing success. Landmark legislation and Supreme Court decisions have established the equal rights of every person, and institutions from schools to businesses have integrated people with disabilities.

"The Americans with Disabilities Act was the Civil Rights Act of civil rights acts," said John Dickerson, executive director of the Arc of Indiana since 1973. "Even up to the '70s, a lot of doctors would say the best thing you could do for the rest of your kids is place them somewhere and forget you ever had them. The movement depended on hotbeds of progressive thought like South Bend and LOGAN, where there were a bunch of dedicated folk who just refused to accept what was.

"Changing culture has transformative moments, but I think it is much more evolutionary than it is revolutionary. Just as bringing kids into the Little Rock schools system was a defining moment, bringing kids into the public schools started a movement. The value of public education is not the skills you learn. It's transmitting the culture."

The grassroots disability movement mirrors the Civil Rights movement. Unlike many other 20th century causes that operate with a top-down model and base their appeal on pity rather than dignity, these two movements gained strength and momentum by promoting the value of all people.

"What's different about the disability movement in many respects is it started first at a local level and grew to a state and a national level," Dickerson said. "It's focused on more change starting on the community level. The real leadership came out of those visionaries back then and still does today. In the '70s and '80s we started talking about respect."

136

Also like the larger Civil Rights movement, the movement in general—and LOGAN in particular—faces a new set of challenges. Its successes suggest to some that an era of special attention has passed and no further progress is required. Tight budgets leave some calculating how to cut resources and services for the disabled. (Dickerson recalls the warning from at least as far back as 1973: "People with disabilities will have rights as long as the middle class can afford it.") A society that will not tolerate racial, ethnic, nor sexist slurs hears "retarded" without wincing, and without the compassion and respect the word evoked on the sign next to LOGAN School.

To meet the challenges, providers continue to unite their voices, advocating for a fair share of resources for people with disabilities through such organizations as INARF, the state trade association representing a coalition of agencies that serves 60,000 people in Indiana and employs more than 14,500. Many of the members are not-for-profit organizations that provide services not available from other sources.

"It's more like a chamber of commerce for this industry. We come up with a unified approach to so many public policy issues," said INARF Director Jim Hammond, who sees the challenges up close. "I don't know how the state would ever be able to respond if tomorrow we had a high incidence of death among those caregivers over 75. How many direct support professionals are out there? What are we doing about the next generation—kids exiting public schools? Who's going to be prepared? Who's going to have the passion and have the skills to operate a blue-chip not-for-profit organization?"

Service challenges result from advocacy successes, as the movement to educate people with disabilities produced more educated, more enlightened parents and children with higher aspirations.

"All the programs like LOGAN started out in the beginning as schools for the retarded," Hammond said. "They evolved into work activity centers after kids aged out. When kids completed their public school, it changed the expectations and aspirations of both the parents and the kids. Parents became more astute and did not accept secondhand services. They needed specialized services."

Within the disability community, a new generation has grown up enjoying the fruits of the pioneers' struggle. Some turn away from the hard-won access to public education and opt for private or home schools. Some withdraw from houses and apartments in ordinary neighborhoods to congregate in exclusive communities behind gates. Some organize around a specific disability in support groups.

While laws have paved the way for inclusion, people still worry about acceptance in a society that places such value on achievement and utility that their child might not meet those measures. Advances in medical technology raise enormous ethical questions for families, with even more likely just over the horizon. What if science develops a genetic or pharmaceutical "cure" for a disability? What would such a life-altering procedure mean for the person? Should it be administered to an adult? A child? An unborn person? What does the answer suggest about "normal," or about personhood itself? What will the world look like without people who function in those ways?

Molly Anderson, whose son KJ has cerebral palsy, believes a narrow view of "normal" would deprive the world of a vital experience of diversity.

"It's based on the foundation that we as a society are blessed to have these people in our lives," she said. "We don't live in a perfect world. You will be better for knowing these people. You will become a better person. You will be better for giving them opportunities. It's allowed me to give more compassion to others, to be more tolerant. I don't think my son looks at people the way the rest of us do. He's different, but he's blind to other people's differences."

We are likely to know before long what the world will look like without Down syndrome children. Prenatal testing and easy access to abortion have dramatically reduced the birth of such children, precisely when a move toward delayed childbearing would have led to a slight increase. Estimates for the rate of abortion for Down syndrome babies range up to 85 percent.

For Kathy Ratkiewicz, a LOGAN parent whose son Danny has Down syndrome, that statistic suggests an exclusion far worse than the out-of-sight, out-of-mind institutionalization of the past: "The biggest disability a lot of these people have is society's attitude. They start out with several strikes against them because people don't think they should be here to start with. The unconditional love is on the part of the person with disabilities. The kids change you."

If the measure of a society is how it treats its weakest members, the response to those with developmental disabilities is a critical yardstick. Concern for a child with autism predicts care for a grandparent with Alzheimer's. Compassion for a birth-injured baby like Rita Jo Newman predicts support for someone who has suffered from an accident. Clearly, solidarity among disabilities is vital to their common claim of equality and infinite human worth. As Martin Luther King warned in the Civil Rights movement: "Injustice anywhere is a threat to justice everywhere."

By those standards, the presence of LOGAN for 60 years has set South Bend apart as a leading-edge location for families who need the services and share the vision of equality. Some business executives have turned down career advancement to stay where their children thrive in an environment of highly skilled service and passionate compassion. Others have left and come back when they discovered the gaps in care elsewhere, including much larger cities.

"LOGAN is an island of excellence," said Steve Fodroczi, who turned down promotion offers in Jacksonville and Los Angeles to keep his son Scott near LOGAN. He and his wife Barbara still volunteer with the agency years after Scott died of cancer.

Throughout the years, LOGAN has been fortunate to have friends in government, advocating on behalf of people with developmental disabilities. One particularly good friend, Joe Kernan, first became involved as a LOGAN volunteer and his wife Maggie as an employee in the 1970s—long before Joe's career took a political path, first as South Bend mayor and eventually as governor of Indiana. Even from the State Capitol, Joe never

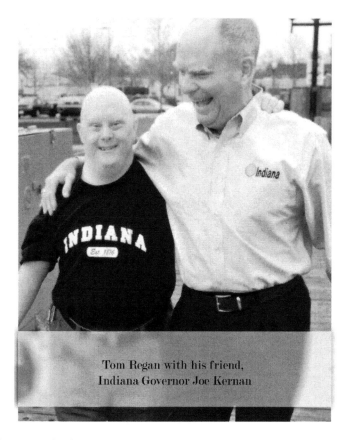

Tom Regan with his friend,
Indiana Governor Joe Kernan

forgot his roots, his home community, or the mission of the agency that introduced him to his good friend Tom Regan, a LOGAN participant. Retired from politics, Joe is now the owner of the South Bend Silver Hawks minor league baseball team. His buddy Tom was one of the first employees Joe hired when he came on board at Covelski Stadium. In August of 2010, his team hosted the first annual LOGAN Night at the Cove with Silver Hawks players partnering with LOGAN players for a three-inning game prior to the actual minor league game that night. LOGAN players were introduced on the field and Dan Harshman threw out the first pitch.

For any movement to maintain its vision, the handoff from the first to the second generation is the most critical. Joe Newman's passion and longevity have kept not only the founders' spirit but also a living founder present for LOGAN. On a visit to South Bend from his Florida retirement home in 2009, at age 96, he pressed the Protective Services Board to find creative ways of enlisting support from others.

But the handoff has been happening for years. When Sally Hamburg was moving from Racine, Wisconsin, to South Bend, a girl in their neighborhood noticed the Jewish symbols on items coming from the van and ran to tell her mother. The mother saw Sally's 18-month-old son Joel, a child with Down syndrome, crawling on the floor and quickly introduced the new neighbor to LOGAN founder Marion Waxman.

"Marion was my mentor," Sally said. "Because of people like Marion, this agency is here. She got me involved in LOGAN. She taught me the way to go about getting the services that were needed for our son. You follow the chain."

Jay Lewis, a lawyer and onetime board chair whose daughter Sarah was born with spina bifida in 1998, said the agency understands itself as a transmitter of the past to the future. "As a board, we have to be careful to keep in mind LOGAN's role as a steward of resources this community has pulled together. There are generations of clients ahead that will need these services. The people in our community are proud of the fact that we collectively have built and maintained this organization. People know that LOGAN is something of a leader in the field. A lot of people participate in small ways. They want to be a part. Everybody has a good feeling about LOGAN. We have to protect that goodwill, too."

Decades after the first informal gathering of parents, Newman, in his dedication speech, called for continuing evolution faithful to the vision of equality and inclusion for all. "Now as I stand here before you, I realize that anything I say in dedication of the building will be an aftermath. That this building has already received its charge, its command, from the LOGANs before it and, yes, through them, the blessings, the hopes, and the desires of all the people who were involved with LOGAN and who have gone before us.

"So I can only borrow words that have been used before. It is now for us, for this community, to dedicate itself to share that commitment with this building, and to continue to protect and preserve the LOGAN saga, and to strengthen its mission.

"LOGAN is a precious stone, to hold and to show with pride. A sturdy precious stone, to be used and treasured, and to be handed down from generation to generation for the benefit of every generation. We must keep it secure. We must keep it polished. We must keep it bright so that it will continue to be a beacon for the people of LOGAN, who are the true treasures of this community."

## Dan Harshman

The word spread quickly in early 1978: LOGAN had hired its Title XX clerk to be its new CEO. Dan Harshman, after just two years with the organization, knew he wasn't its first, or even second, choice for the leadership role. He embraced the job anyway. Today, his leadership of the leading-edge organization wins broad admiration.

"I still feel so tied to the people that hired me and what they wanted," Harshman said. "LOGAN had this great history and these great people. I kind of learned at their knee which gave me the desire to understand what they wanted and what they stood for. We've always been one of the state leaders in the field."

Harshman, a running back on Notre Dame's 1966 championship team under Coach Ara Parseghian, first connected to people with developmental disabilities as a student volunteer at NISH—the state institution for children next door to where LOGAN Center would eventually be built and Dan would begin his career. After graduation, he went on to teach junior high English in New York and served as a juvenile parole officer in Toledo, Ohio, where he learned that he liked the not-for-profit world.

At LOGAN, where he signed on to oversee the details of Title XX funding, he quickly became responsible for leading-edge efforts that

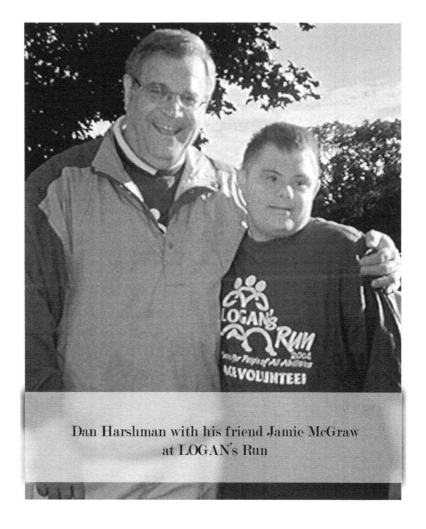

**Dan Harshman with his friend Jamie McGraw
at LOGAN's Run**

ranged from winning state grants to suing state agencies, closing unsatisfactory institutions to opening group homes in neighborhoods.

"We would speak up on issues, we'd step out on issues," he said. "I think LOGAN always wanted to listen to a consumer voice and start things, get things going."

Almost as soon as he took the CEO position, he was involved in approaching state legislators at the capitol for money to build a new LOGAN Industries.

"At the time it was the largest workshop grant," Harshman recalled. "That helped me get some confidence. It's a whole different world working around government down there. The legislative side is so different from the administrative side. That grant helped us get something planted that was real. We got to build LOGAN Industries, and that was exciting."

Since then, Harshman has overseen LOGAN's expansion—a far greater than anticipated role for Protective Services, group homes and other residential settings, high-profile activities in the community, building two new facilities, launching the Regional Autism Center.

After four years of preparing for the 1987 International Summer Special Olympics, Harshman found himself sidelined, looking after an Irish athlete and his family when the young man was hospitalized after a seizure led to an injury that left him unconscious and eventually proved fatal. "That was my whole week," he recalled.

After the event, he leveraged the intense community attention on LOGAN, establishing the agency among the premier charitable organizations in town and hiring Ann Lagomarcino to manage first the volunteers and then the marketing.

Through it all, Harshman has held together LOGAN's sometimes crosscurrent dedication to advocacy and services.

"By doing both, we are stronger, more effective, and make a farther reaching impact," he says. "By caring about the issues, we're a better provider. We're a better advocate because we're not riding in on our white horse.

"The parents on the board didn't just care about their kid. That has been the strength behind LOGAN. The parents advocated for all the kids. They understood that caring about all of LOGAN would benefit not only their sons and daughters but future families as well. This basic understanding that our founders had is one that must be encouraged in today's families."

## Dear LOGAN Friends & Families:

It was not easy writing this book, trying to put to paper the vibrant story of LOGAN. Sixty years of memories is a long time. Though many memories remain colorful and vivid, I know that we have just scratched the surface of the tales that make up the LOGAN Story.

Countless volunteers have given their time, talent, and energy—serving on boards and committees, working at events, and befriending individuals with disabilities. Countless donors as well as community businesses, organizations, and individual leaders have shown their support of our mission in so many ways. Countless staff have gone the extra mile to add quality to the lives of the people who count on them. Countless parents, guardians, and family members have shown us the way to care for those they love. And, countless individuals with disabilities have opened our hearts and our minds to true potential.

LOGAN's history is a blend of so many heartwarming stories of people who cared enough to dream, to hope, and to work to make this community welcoming to all who call it home. Whether you are directly part of LOGAN or part of a similar community elsewhere, it is likely that your own personal story is mirrored in the stories told here.

LOGAN has prospered in a community, a state, and a country that have embraced our mission. It has never been easy, and never will be, to raise awareness and money, to create new services and laws or to correct injustices. LOGAN's story is a tribute to our founders. They likely never imagined that their hard work, positive spirit, and belief in the cause would lead to such incredible results. Yet, these very same founders would be the first to remind us that there is always more to be done. They knew back then what we now know—the torch must be passed.

Sincerely,

Dan Harshman
Chief Executive Officer
LOGAN Community Resources, Inc.

# Appendix

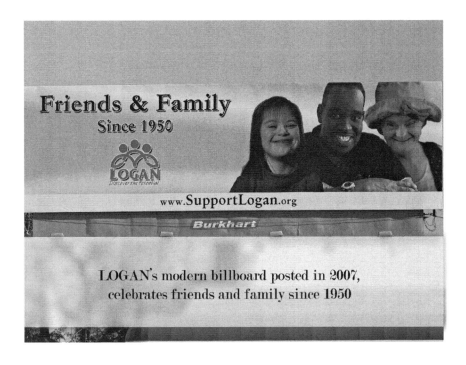

LOGAN's modern billboard posted in 2007, celebrates friends and family since 1950

# The Movement

## 1950s
## The Beginnings—getting families and the community to believe

| Year | LOGAN | State and National |
|------|-------|--------------------|
| 1950 | The Council for the Retarded of St. Joseph County is incorporated | The Arc of the United States is founded |
| 1951 | LOGAN School opens on Logan Street in Mishawaka with 22 students/2 teachers | |
| 1954 | | Catalyst of Civil Rights Movement—*Brown v. Board of Education of Topeka.* U.S. Supreme Court rules separate schools as unequal and unconstitutional |
| 1955 | Adult Training Program (LOGAN Industries) begins | |
| 1956 | LOGAN is approved for United Way funds | The Arc of Indiana is founded |

## 1960s
## Laying the groundwork for the right
## to education and work

| Year | LOGAN | State and National |
|------|-------|--------------------|
| 1961 | First executive director, Myron Birkey, is hired | President John F. Kennedy appoints a special President's Panel on Mental Retardation |
| 1964 | | Civil Rights Act signed by President Lyndon B. Johnson |
| 1965 | | Medicare and Medicaid established by passing of Social Security Amendments |
| 1966 | LOGAN Industries moves to High Street (former South Bend Tackle Building) | The President's Committee on Mental Retardation established by President Johnson |
| 1969 | New LOGAN Center is built and opens on Eddy Street, across from University of Notre Dame | President's Committee on Mental Retardation conference introduces normalization concept |

## 1970s
## An explosion of advocacy and services

| Year | LOGAN | State and National |
|------|-------|--------------------|
| 1970 | HomeStart—early intervention program for children from birth to 5 years begins. | |
| 1972 | National Center for Law and the Handicapped, founded by Notre Dame and LOGAN, launches as first U.S. legal advocacy center for people with disabilities<br><br>Northern Indiana State Hospital (NISH) remains open after outpouring of family and community support | Parents of residents of Willow Brook State School (Staten Island, NY) file lawsuit to end appalling conditions; Public outrage triggered by TV broadcast from facility; Eventually, thousands are moved to community |
| 1973 | First Adult Rehabilitation classroom opens, serving individuals with severe disabilities | Rehabilitation Act passes, outlawing exclusion and discrimination of people with disabilities from programs receiving federal funds |
| 1974 | LOGAN Protective Services Board is established | *Halderman v. Pennhurst* filed; Pennhurst State School and Hospital (PA) conditions exposed; Precedent for deinstitutionalization and right to community services<br><br>Indiana Association of Rehabilitation Facilities (INARF) founded; Costa Miller, first director, holds position for 30 years |

151

## 1970s (continued)
## An explosion of advocacy and services

| Year | LOGAN | State and National |
|------|-------|--------------------|
| 1975 | | Education of All Handicapped Children Act mandates free and appropriate public education in least restrictive environment; eventually re-named IDEA (The Individuals With Disabilities Act) |
| 1977 | Title XX funding crisis at LOGAN averted after out-pouring of community support | |

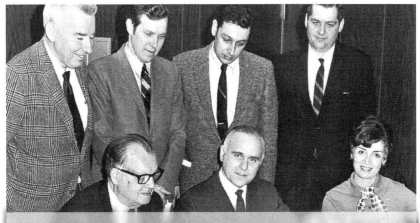

LOGAN Board Members, 1968
Top Row: Joe Doyle, Leonard Whitfield, Harvey Bender
and Edward Kalamaros
Bottom Row: Dick Gamble, Erv Derda and Mary Ann Matthews

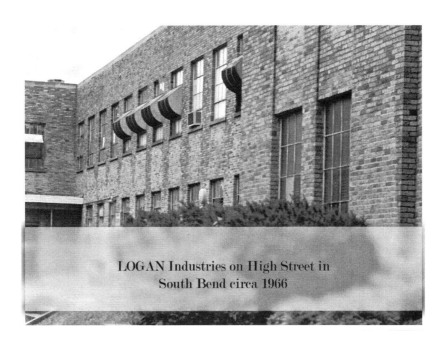

LOGAN Industries on High Street in
South Bend circa 1966

## 1980s
## Keeping mission top of mind and preparing
## for life in the community

| Year | LOGAN | State and National |
|------|-------|--------------------|
| 1981 | New LOGAN Industries on Boland Drive opens | International Year of Disabled Persons is launched<br><br>Parents of "Baby Doe"—Bloomington, IN—advised to decline surgery to newborn with Down syndrome; disability rights activists intervened; baby dies before legal action taken |
| 1983 | LOGAN purchases first group home | |
| 1986 | Employment Services Program begins for community work<br><br>Semi-Independent Living Program launches, supporting people in apartments and homes | Legislation passed creating P & A (Protection & Advocacy agencies) |
| 1987 | International Summer Special Olympics Games are held on the campuses of Notre Dame and Saint Mary's College | |
| 1988 | LOGAN Foundation Board is started and endowment fund is established | |
| 1989 | LOGAN opens ninth group home, all agency-owned<br><br>The Great LOGAN Nose-On is launched, becoming agency's signature community awareness and fundraising event | Congressional Task Force on Rights and Empowerment of Americans with Disabilities is created, beginning grass roots support for Americans with Disabilities Act (ADA) |

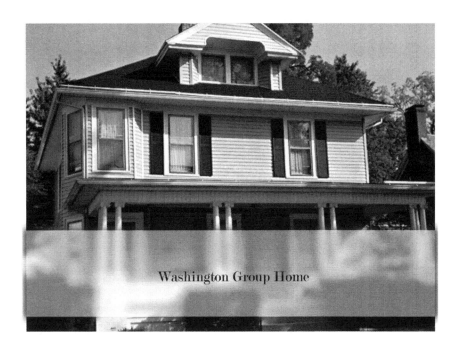

Washington Group Home

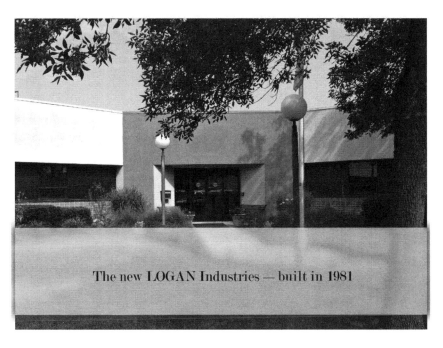

The new LOGAN Industries — built in 1981

## 1990s
## A time of increased exposure and fundraising

| Year | LOGAN | State and National |
|------|-------|--------------------|
| 1990 | | President George H. W. Bush signs Americans with Disabilities Act (ADA), providing civil rights protection for those with disabilities |
| 1991 | LOGAN begins use of Medicaid Waiver funds to start Community Living pilot program, supporting people in their own apartments and homes | First Steps and Special Education pre-schools established |
| 1993 | LOGAN achieves accreditation through CARF (Commission on Accreditation of Rehabilitation Facilities)— accreditation continues to be maintained | |
| 1997 | Organization's name is officially changed from Council for the Retarded of St. Joseph County to LOGAN Community Resources, Inc. | Indiana adopts 317 Plan, refocusing state efforts to close state hospitals for people with developmental disabilities and allocating $40 million new dollars to further develop community-based services |
| 1999 | LOGAN receives first Leighton Award for Non-Profit Excellence from the Community Foundation, awarding a $100,000 gift to be matched for the recipient's endowment fund | Supreme Court decides in Olmstead case that individuals with disabilities must be offered services in most integrated setting possible; legal precedent for future actions to help people move to community setting; leads way for LOGAN's class action lawsuit |

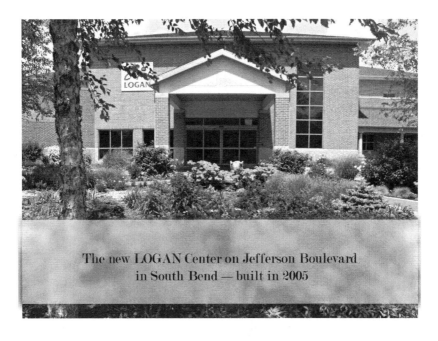

The new LOGAN Center on Jefferson Boulevard
in South Bend — built in 2005

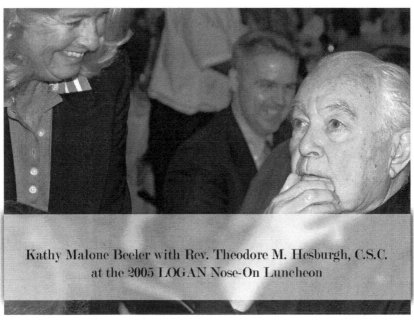

Kathy Malone Beeler with Rev. Theodore M. Hesburgh, C.S.C.
at the 2005 LOGAN Nose-On Luncheon

## 2000s
## Major steps continue with partnership increasing

| Year | LOGAN | State and National |
|------|-------|--------------------|
| 2001 | Jefferson Boulevard property donated by Saint Joseph Regional Medical Center | |
| 2002 | LOGAN's Run is launched as a major community event and fundraiser | Betty Williams, co-president of Self Advocates of Indiana, travels to Japan to represent self-advocates from the U.S. |
| 2003 | LOGAN files class action lawsuit (*Kraus v. Hamilton*), filed on behalf of 1,600 people with developmental disabilities living in nursing homes | |
| 2004 | LOGAN connects with community partners to launch Regional Autism Center; LOGAN assumes fundraising and operational responsibility | Dr. David Braddock issues report on Indiana's progress in funding and services in the community |
| 2005 | LOGAN Center on Jefferson Boulevard opens | |
| 2006 | Regional Autism Center is renamed the *Sonya Ansari Center for Autism at LOGAN* | The UN General Assembly Center adopts Convention on the Rights of Persons with Disabilities |
| 2007 | | Fort Wayne State Developmental Center closes, marking the end of Indiana's institutions for individuals with developmental disabilities |

# Historical Snapshot

|                                                                       | 1950     | 2010          |
|-----------------------------------------------------------------------|----------|---------------|
| Number of families served by LOGAN                                    | 22       | 1,200         |
| Number of LOGAN employees                                             | 2        | 370           |
| Annual budget                                                         | $10,500  | $14,642,000   |
| State and federal funding for community based services                | $0       | $876,935,737  |
| Number of individuals living in large state hospitals in Indiana      | 4,713    | 0             |
| Number of children in special education classes in Indiana public schools | 0    | 210, 733      |
| St. Joseph County organizations serving people with developmental disabilities | 1 | 20          |

# Governmental Partners

Government has been an increasingly involved partner for legislation
and funding for people with developmental disabilities.
These partners have been very important to advocacy
and service expansion.

State of Indiana
First Steps
FSSA (Family and Social Services Administration)
BDDS (Bureau of Developmental Disabilities Services)
Governors
State Representatives
State Senators
St. Joseph County Council
St. Joseph County Prosecutor's Office
City of Mishawaka
City of South Bend

# State Associations

These state associations have spearheaded growth in services
and awareness in Indiana

**Arc of Indiana**
Founded 1956—John Dickerson, Executive Director, since 1983

**Indiana University/Indiana Institute on Disability and Community**
Founded 1971—Dr. David Mank, Director, since 1981

**Indiana Resource Center for Autism**,
affiliate of Indiana Institute on Disability and Community
Dr. Cathy Pratt, Director, since 1994

**Indiana Association of Rehabilitation Facilities (INARF)**
Founded 1974—Costa Miller, Director (1974-2004)
Jim Hammond, President and CEO, since 2004

# Community Partners

LOGAN has not been alone in creating services and opportunities.
Our founding parents knew early on that partners were critical to the
success of what they were trying to accomplish.
The list of community organizations that have offered ongoing services
and support to LOGAN's mission continues to grow.

Bethel College
Center for the Homeless
Community Foundation of
    St. Joseph County
Daughters of Isabella
Family and Children's Center
Holy Cross College
Hospice of St. Joseph County
Indiana University South Bend
Joint Services for Special Education for School City of Mishawaka/
    Penn-Harris-Madison
    School Corporation
Junior League of South Bend

Knights of Columbus
Madison Center
Memorial Hospital
REAL Services
Saint Mary's College
Service Guild
South Bend Community School
    Corporation
South Bend Heritage Foundation
Saint Joseph Regional Medical Center
United Way of St. Joseph County
University of Notre Dame
YMCA
YWCA

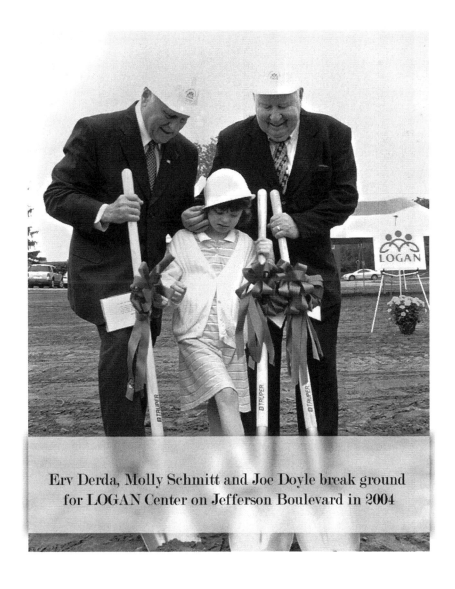

Erv Derda, Molly Schmitt and Joe Doyle break ground
for LOGAN Center on Jefferson Boulevard in 2004

# Peer Providers

In a community of our size, LOGAN is fortunate to have so many
outstanding organizations serving and supporting people with disabilities.
Back in 1950, LOGAN was the only local provider
for services for people with developmental disabilities.
As more families came forward and the need grew,
other local organizations sprang up to provide services.
This is a measure of how far our community and
surrounding areas have come in support of people with disabilities.

ADEC
AWS
Camp Millhouse
Cardinal Center
Challenger Little League
Chiara Home
Children's Dispensary
Corvilla
Dungarvin
Foundation for Music and Healing
Forte Residential, Inc.
Globe Star
Goodwill Industries
Hannah and Friends
Help at Home
In-Pact
In*Source/Parent Information
    Center
Indiana Mentor
Joint Educational Services and
    Special Education
Marshall Starke Development
    Center
MDC Goldenrod
Michiana Down Syndrome
    Family and Advocacy Group
Michiana Resources
Mosaic
Opportunity Enterprises
Partners in Opportunities
Reins of Life
ResCare, Inc.
Sam-Lin
SHARE Foundation
S.O.L.O. Ski Program
Special Olympics of
    St. Joseph County

# LOGAN Staff

The staff at LOGAN is so important in the lives of the people served.
In their own unique ways, these staff members have contributed to the
mission of LOGAN, making a difference in the lives of many people.

### PRESENT STAFF WITH OVER 30 YEARS OF SERVICE

| | | |
|---|---|---|
| Tim Silverberg | Community Habilitation Instructor | 38 years |
| Debra Beach | Director, Service Coordination | 35 years |
| John Ayers | Sales Manager, LOGAN Industries | 34 years |

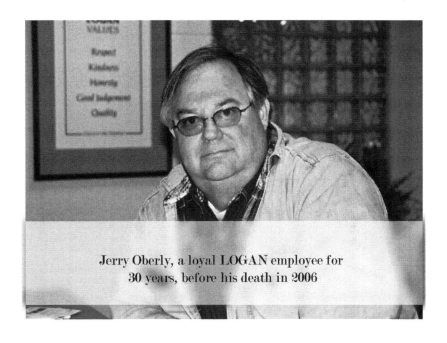

Jerry Oberly, a loyal LOGAN employee for
30 years, before his death in 2006

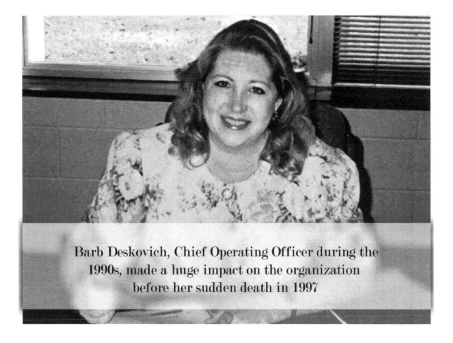

Barb Deskovich, Chief Operating Officer during the
1990s, made a huge impact on the organization
before her sudden death in 1997

| Dan Harshman | Chief Executive Officer | 34 years |
| Herb Johnson | Maintenance Worker | 33 years |
| Jane Schmidt | Occupational Therapist/Building Blocks and *Sonya Ansari* Center for Autism | 33 years |
| Bill Kring | Program Assistant, Supported Living | 32 years |
| Dan Ryan | Director, *Sonya Ansari* Center for Autism | 32 years |
| Marilyn Florey | Caseworker, LOGAN Protective Services | 31 years |

## PRESENT STAFF WITH OVER 20 YEARS OF SERVICE

| Gail Eastman | Caseworker, LOGAN Protective Services | 28 years |
| Reeney Poinsette | Developmental Therapist, Building Blocks | 27 years |
| Jenny Crowe Demske | Service Coordinator | 26 years |
| Brenda Kulp | Habilitation Instructor, LOGAN Industries | 26 years |
| Margaret Mathews | Customer Service Manager, LOGAN Industries | 26 years |
| Ann Georgia | Administrative Assistant, Group Living | 25 years |
| Annie Micinski | Service Coordinator | 25 years |
| Char Geary | Developmental Therapist, Building Blocks | 24 years |
| Susan Correa | Caseworker, Protective Services | 23 years |
| Ann Lagomarcino | Director of Marketing | 22 years |
| Londa Miltenberger | Team Coordinator, Adult Day Services | 22 years |
| Faye White | Employee Benefits Manager, Human Resources | 21 years |
| Peg Leonardo | Developmental Therapist, Building Blocks | 21 years |
| Jan Seago | Developmental Therapist, Building Blocks | 21 years |
| Cherry Silverberg | Nurse, Adult Day Services | 21 years |
| Cheri Sauer | Administrative Assistant, Building Blocks | 20 years |
| Roshonda White | Program Assistant, Supported Living | 20 years |

## FORMER STAFF WITH OVER 30 YEARS OF SERVICE

| Vern Batten | Maintenance |
| John Fischers | LOGAN Industries |
| Jerry Oberly | Director, Maintenance and Housekeeping |
| Dorinda Rupe | LOGAN Protective Services |

## FORMER STAFF WITH OVER 20 YEARS OF SERVICE

| Bob Bastock | LOGAN Industries |
| Marilyn Casper | Building Blocks |
| Evelyn Feder | LOGAN Industries |
| Margaret Garvey | LOGAN Protective Services |
| Becky Mahl | Service Coordination |

Leeann Rappelli     Adult Day Services
Anne Rohr     Employment Services
Brad Stahoviak     LOGAN Industries

## LOGAN INITIAL STAFF/EXECUTIVE DIRECTORS

| | | |
|---|---|---|
| Ada Marker | 1951 | First Teacher |
| Charles Gesslein | 1957 | First Principal |
| Myron Birkey | 1961-1964 | First Executive Director |
| Richard Rembold | 1964-1965 | Executive Director |
| Myron Birkey | 1965-1968 | Executive Director |
| Robert Wesjahn | 1968-1970 | Executive Director |
| Linden Thorn | 1970-1973 | Executive Director |
| Aloysius Soenneker | 1974-1977 | Executive Director |
| Jack Greeley | 1977-1978 | Acting Executive Director |
| Dan Harshman | 1978— | Chief Executive Officer |

## LOGAN CORPORATE BOARD PRESIDENTS

| | |
|---|---|
| Joseph J. Newman | 1950-1951 |
| Fr. James Smythe | 1952-1954 |
| Marion Waxman | 1955-1956 |
| Lloyd Pieratt | 1957-1958 |
| Martha Abernethy | 1959-1960 |
| Dick Gamble | 1961-1964 |
| Joe Doyle | 1965-1969 |
| Erv Derda | 1970-1973 |
| Dick Cleary | 1974-1979 |
| John Burgess | 1980-1982 |
| Steve Fodroczi | 1983-1984 |
| Vince O'Connor | 1985-1986 |
| Sally Hamburg | 1987-1988 |
| Howard Mueller | 1989-1990 |
| Ralph Komasinski | 1991-1992 |
| Steve Pajakowski | 1993-1994 |
| Brian Hay | 1995-1996 |
| Cathy Wynne | 1997-1998 |
| Kevin Kelly | 1999-2000 |
| Bob King | 2001-2003 |
| Pat Pinnick | 2004-2005 |
| Jay Lewis | 2006-2007 |
| Pam von Rahl | 2008-2009 |
| John Firth | 2010— |

## LOGAN PROTECTIVE SERVICES BOARD PRESIDENTS

| | |
|---|---|
| Joseph J. Newman | 1974-1977 |
| Jim Farris | 1978-1979 |
| Tom Merluzzi, Ph.D. | 1980-1982 |
| Barbara O'Connor | 1983-1984 |
| Marcia Lemay | 1985-1986 |
| Tom Spencer | 1987-1989 |
| Carol Ann Mooney | 1990-1991 |
| Alberta Barnes | 1992 |
| Dr. Dick Reineke | 1993-1994 |
| Fran McDonald | 1995-1999 |
| Margot Reagan | 2000-2004 |
| Tony Ashbaugh | 2005 |
| Anne Kellenberg-True | 2006 |
| Brandon Zabukovic | 2007-2009 |
| Jay Lewis | 2010— |

## LOGAN FOUNDATION BOARD PRESIDENTS

| | |
|---|---|
| Erv Derda | 1989-1991 |
| Gene Cavanaugh | 1992-1993 |
| Abe Marcus | 1994-1995 |
| Dick Mellinger | 1996-1997 |
| Fr. Bill Beauchamp | 1989-1999 |
| Mary Jane Stanley | 2000-2001 |
| Ben Ziolkowski | 2002-2003 |
| Kathy Malone Beeler | 2004-2005 |
| Leo Ditchcreek | 2006-2007 |
| Mike Seamon | 2008-2009 |
| Lori Skora | 2010— |

# About the Author

Gene Stowe, a freelance writer based in South Bend, Indiana, grew up in the Carolinas, graduated from the University of North Carolina at Chapel Hill and earned a Master of Theological Studies degree from Trinity Seminary in Columbus, Ohio. He was a reporter for The Charlotte (NC) Observer for 13 years before he moved to South Bend, where he taught at Trinity School at Greenlawn for 15 years. He developed and implemented the writing program and the religion program at the school.

Stowe, who has six grown children, returned to full-time writing in 2007 and produces newspaper and magazine articles, web copy, marketing material, speeches, and books for a variety of clients, including the *South Bend Tribune*, the College of Science at the University of Notre Dame, and *Racing Toward Diversity* magazine. He also provides tutoring and consulting services in English and writing. He is a principal in Write Smack Dab LLC and the author of the nonfiction narrative *Inherit the Land: Jim Crow Meets Miss Maggie's Will*, published in 2006 by the University Press of Mississippi.

LOGAN is a community organization which provides advocacy, services, and resources for children and adults with developmental disabilities. Since 1950, LOGAN has been here for families, expanding to meet changing needs through ventures like the *Sonya Ansari* Center for Autism. Now reaching over 1,200 families each year, LOGAN provides a full range of services from therapies and specialty camps for children to employment, training, recreation, and community living options for teens and adults. At the very heart of LOGAN is advocacy which fuels our work within the community to increase resources and opportunities for people with disabilities.

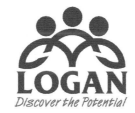

2505 E. Jefferson Boulevard
South Bend, IN 46615
(574) 289-4831

Visit our websites
www.logancenter.org
www.loganindustries.com
www.ansaricenterforautism.org

To order additional copies of
# voice
**disability and ability at LOGAN, 1950-2010**
Call LOGAN or visit www.logancenter.org